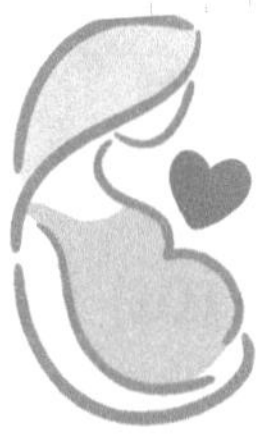

Pregnancy Diary

A must for every mom-to-be

Bakul Raut

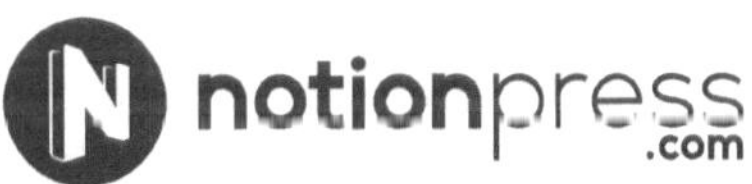

Notion Press

Old No. 38, New No. 6
McNichols Road, Chetpet
Chennai - 600 031

First Published by Notion Press 2018
Copyright © Bakul Raut 2018
All Rights Reserved.

ISBN 978-1-64429-061-3

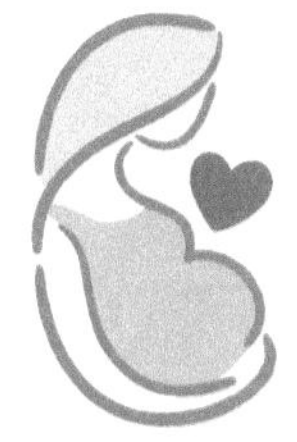

This
Pregnancy Diary
belongs to

MOTHER ___________________

FATHER ___________________

DOCTOR ___________________

DUE DATE ___________________

EMERGENCY NOS. ___________________

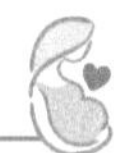

Congratulations on owning this Pregnancy Diary which would be a great companion for you during this beautiful journey of motherhood.

The contents of this diary are intended solely to make available general summarized information to expecting mothers and their families. This diary should not be substituted for medical advice. You must consult your doctor before acting on anything presented in this diary.

The best use of this diary would be to gain knowledge alongside your experiences of motherhood, rather than personalize the content for your self-experienced situations.

Every woman is unique and so is her pregnancy.

Use the notes in the diary to write questions and doubts you may have in mind, to ask your doctor on your next visit. There is no substitute to your doctor. Not even this diary.

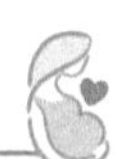

TOPIC	PAGE

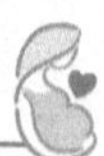

 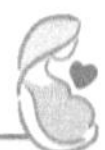

Being a mother makes every woman complete. It is the beginning of life afresh with a new perspective to it. It is the joy of oneness and the sense of belonging to the one who is going to exist because of you.

As you go into this beautiful journey of motherhood, life will change, with every passing day and week. Changes that would make you excited, intense, concerned, curious and sometimes furious as well. There is a reason for every change that you experience as a new life is beginning to exist with you. You have to now care for yourself and your baby as well!

This diary is a compilation of most of the events that would occur to you and your baby, the do's and don'ts that you will have to adhere to, the nutrition that would be the best for you and the answers to most questions you may have. This diary is an essential tool that guides through the various changes that happen to you and within you.

Every pregnancy is as unique as you are, and hence, no general guidelines apply at par for all. Use this diary to gain knowledge about your baby and yourself and make this experience of motherhood easier to absorb. Do not personalize the contents of this diary for your self-experienced situations, as the best advisor to all your experiences still remains your doctor.

This diary guides you from week 6 up to week 40 of pregnancy. Do not be in a hurry to jump to the forthcoming weeks and know things in advance. Rather, make this diary your companion till the baby is born and refer to only the week that you are currently on. This will be a joyful read as you explore the changes happening to and within you.

Highlight, underline, comment or simply doodle in the diary whenever you find yourself in a situation mentioned in it.

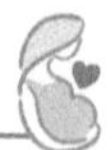

This can be an interesting memoir to look back at in the growing years of your baby.

During your pregnancy, you would imagine your baby. Be it boy or girl, you would start building your dreams around the baby. Start writing names for baby boy or baby girl in the diary as it is difficult to recollect a good name that you liked and had thought of earlier. After baby is born, you can select the name you would like from the one's you have already listed.

Regular doctor visits are a must for the well being of both you and your baby. Make entries in the doctor visit schedule and do not forget to mention the reason, be it a routine visit or a discomfort that made you visit your doctor. This schedule table would be a good reference as you progress into your pregnancy.

Not all moms-to-be remember all the questions they wanted to ask when they visit the doctor. Do write all the questions and observations that you would like to bring to your doctor's notice when you visit next in the notes.

This diary also provides space for some special notes or instructions that your doctor may like you to know. Ask your doctor to enter his or her notes too.

I hope this diary would be useful to you and wish you and your baby joy and happiness forever.

BABY GIRL NAMES

BABY BOY NAMES

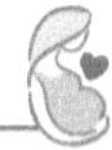

Visit Date	Next Visit	Reason

DOCTOR VISIT SCHEDULE 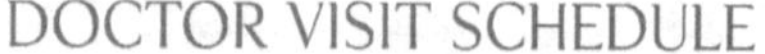

Visit Date	Next Visit	Reason

NOTES

NOTES

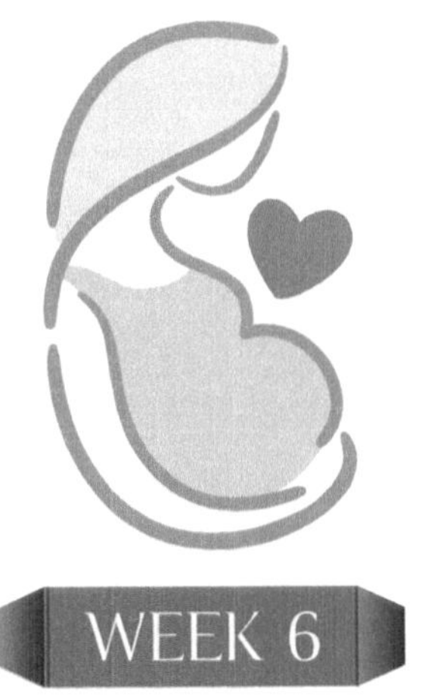

WEEK 6

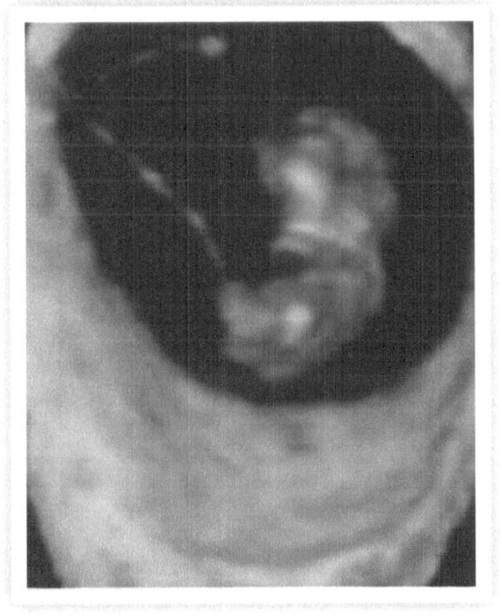

FOETUS AGE 4 WEEKS

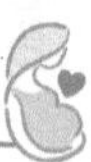

Changes in Baby

- From crown to rump, your baby measures at 2-4 mm or 0.08-0.16 inch - the size of a small lentil.

- This week marks the beginning of the embryonic period which spans from the 6th to 10th weeks of pregnancy or the 4th to 8th week of fetal development.

- Growth is rapid this week with your baby resembling a tadpole with a tail but no brain.

- It is already 10,000 times larger than the fertilized egg; it doesn't have gender characteristics yet.

- Over the next 5 months, more than 100 billion neurons will be formed in the brain, laying the necessary groundwork for a lifetime of learning.

- The baby's heart, the size of poppy seed, is beating on its own.

- Your baby at this stage has it's own bloodstream with blood circulating already.

- Testes or ovaries at this stage are mere clusters of cells.

- Other major organs continue to develop; including liver, kidneys and lungs.

- The head has the beginnings of the eyes, ears and mouth and there are tiny buds which will become arms and legs.

Changes in You

- You may have gained few kilos by now; conversely due to not eating well and nausea, you may have lost some weight.

- In first time pregnancies, abdominal changes are not that apparent.

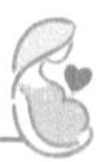

- Changes in breasts are obvious for some. Breasts may feel full and tender and the nipples already more prominent now.

- Aerolas darken to brownish circles of patches around the nipples.

- Bluish veins may be seen just under the skin as the blood supply to breasts increases.

- If you have a pelvic exam, your doctor can usually feel your uterus and note some change in it's size.

- The pregnancy hormone hCG continues to increase, making you prone to fatigue and nausea.

- You may find yourself noticing babies more and wondering how yours will look.

- Your may find yourself thinking a lot about how your life will change, now that you are pregnant. You will probably start thinking about a wardrobe change if you are pregnant for the first time. In other words, your appearance is probably going to occupy your mind in a different way.

Good to Know

Definitions of time

- *Gestational age (menstrual age)* – begins from the 1st day of your last menstrual period (LMP), about 2 weeks before you conceive. This age is mostly used by doctors for calculation purposes. Average length of pregnancy is 40 weeks.

- *Ovulatory age (fertilization age)* – begins the day you conceive. Average length of pregnancy is 38 weeks.

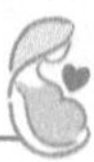

- *Fetal age* – the actual age of the growing fetus (always 2 weeks behind gestational age).

- *Trimester* – each trimester consists of 13 weeks. There are 3 trimesters in pregnancy.

- *Lunar months* – a pregnancy lasts an average of 10 lunar months (28 days each) hence 280 days in total.

Due date calculation

- It doesn't matter when you think you became pregnant. Your doctor will calculate your due date from the first day of your last menstrual period (LMP).

- The main reason being many women don't know for sure when they ovulated. Your doctor will use the LMP as an equalizer to deal with the variations in cycles of every pregnant woman to reach the same calendar.

- For instance, if your LMP was 20th February, your due date will be calculated thus: 7 + 20 and minus 3 months i.e. your due date will be 27th November.

Wholesome Advice

- If you do consume alcohol, stay away from it from the moment your pregnancy is confirmed. Don't kid yourself into thinking an occasional drink is fine. It is tricky knowing the safe levels of consumption. Hence, please stay away from alcohol completely.

- Start saving now for maternity clothes; they can be expensive.

- Your baby is totally, completely dependent on you for all it's needs. To ensure it gets a proper headstart in life, it is important that you eat right, rest enough and stay as healthy as possible throughout your pregnancy.

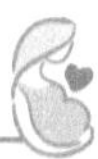

Your Actions Can Impact Your Baby's Growth

Heartburn

- Progesterone causes the burning sensation in the middle of your chest or upper digestive tract. This hormone relaxes the muscle that is responsible for controlling the opening at the top of the stomach.

- Secondly, progesterone causes the stomach to empty more slowly so that as many nutrients as possible can be absorbed from the food you eat. The stomach gets compressed as you grow bigger. It may begin early, although it tends to become more severe later in pregnancy.

- Avoid sodium bicarbonate (baking soda) as it contains a lot of salt which will cause water retention.

- Avoid fatty and greasy foods, carbonated drinks, processed meats and junk food.

- Eat slowly. The more slowly you eat, the more time the enzymes in your saliva will have to break down the food before it reaches your stomach.

- Eat in the correct proportions; heartburn is more likely to flare up if you overfill, in particular with carbohydrates. Don't eat too close to bedtime.

- Avoid lying flat on your back when you are resting or sleeping as this intensifies heartburn. Try propping yourself up on pillows.

- Check with your doctor on antacids.

Stress

- A major change, including a happy one, is stressful. You will read that stress is bad for your baby - this thought

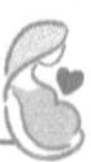

alone is going to stress you out. A reassuring fact to know is millions of healthy and happy babies are born each year to mothers who were stressed out, including in early pregnancy. So, don't stress over the fact that you are stressed!

- Of course, attempts to de-stress should be made if you are overly stressed; anything in excess is no good.

Common Concerns

Whom can I talk to about my fears and concerns while I am pregnant?

- It is important to establish a sound relationship with your doctor so that you can ask him or her anything about your condition. Your doctor knows you, your history and what has happened in the course of your pregnancy so far. Do not hesitate to discuss your doubts and worries with your doctor. Expand on your knowledge by reading good articles and books.

I feel embarrassed discussing some issues with my doctor as they seem silly or trivial.

- Do not be afraid to ask your doctor even on the minor things or be concerned about how he or she will react. Your doctor may have already heard the question before, so don't let that inhibit you. It is their role to clear your doubts. Smallest details should be raised as they can pose risks. So unless you find out, you may never know. Prepare your lists and discuss them during your appointments.

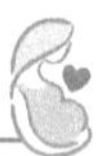

Nutrition

- You must be selective in your meal choices. You cannot just eat whatever you want these days. You are after all eating for two, in terms of quality and quantity.

- Eating the right foods in the right amounts requires planning. Eat foods high in iron, calcium, magnesium, folic acid and zinc.

- You also need fiber and fluids to help solve any constipation problems.

- Foods to help your baby grow and develop include:
    - Bread, cereal, pasta and rice
    - Fruits and vegetables
    - Meat or other protein sources
    - Dairy products
    - Fats, sweets and other 'empty' calorie foods

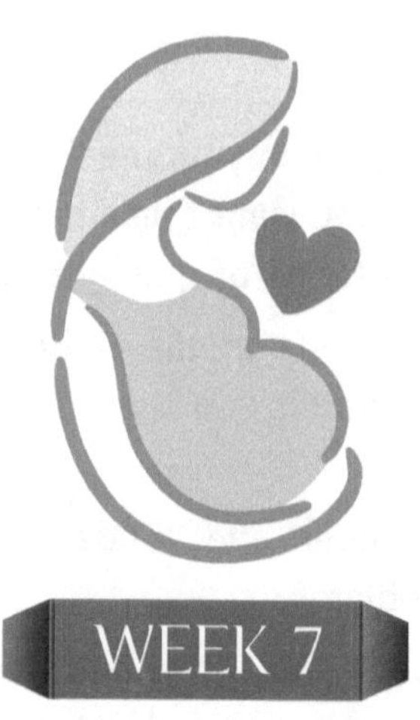

WEEK 7

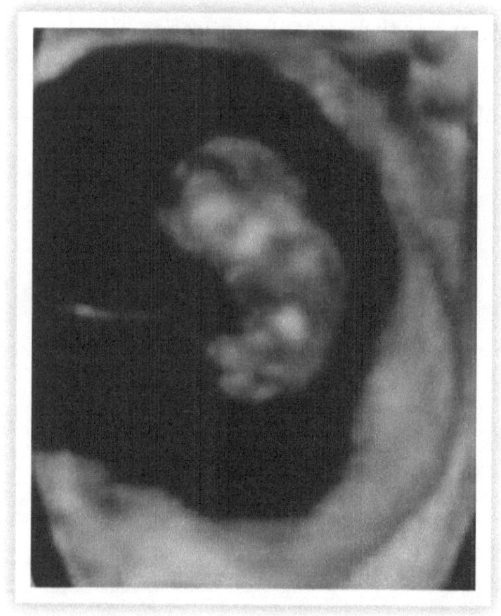

FOETUS AGE 5 WEEKS

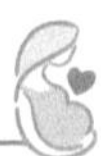

Changes in Baby

- From crown to rump, at the start of the week your baby measures at 4-5 mm or 0.16-0.2 inch, the size of a small raspberry.

- This week your baby goes through an incredible growth spurt.

- Intestines are developing, the heart chambers are forming and the brain hemispheres are growing.

- Other changes are the dark spots where the eyes and the nostrils are to be, are forming; the color in the irises are now visible and the lenses of the baby's eyes are forming.

- Pits that mark the ears and protruding buds that will eventually become the arms and legs begin to appear.

- The appendix is now present along with the pancreas.

- The skull is still transparent and the baby's brain is continuing in its venture to become more complex.

Changes in You

- If you were to have an ultrasound now, it would be able to detect the beating heart of the baby.

- Changes are gradual - you still won't show and many can't tell you are pregnant.

- Weight gain is very slow, covering all parts of your body.

- Your blood pressure is lower, than it was before you got pregnant.

- Some women may even lose weight due to nausea - this is not unusual nor something to worry about. Weight gain in the first trimester is not as important as in the subsequent trimesters when baby goes through major growth and development.

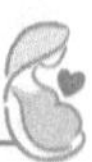

- Pregnancy symptoms like nausea, fatigue, etc. are to be expected in this time period.

- By the 7th week the mucus plug is well established in your cervix; its function is to block out germs and prevent infections. The plug loses and passes in preparation for labor.

- While you may be elated you cannot help but feel anxious and fearful at the prospect of becoming a mother.

- During this phase you will have dreams and fantasies about what your baby will be like - these are the beginnings of your emotional bond with your unborn child.

Good to Know

hCG Hormone

- During weeks 6 and 7, the hCG hormone (manufactured by the placenta) which was responsible for the positive sign during your pregnancy test, may have now built up enough to trigger another change - morning sickness!

- Many women start to feel nauseated, total exhaustion, queasy and generally lousy.

- Morning sickness is just a misnomer - it can happen at any time of the day. Nausea and vomiting are signs of a healthy pregnancy. If you don't have these symptoms, the opposite isn't true. You are just plain lucky.

- Nausea does not affect the baby. Right now they are tiny, so they don't have huge nutritional demands.

- So even if you are not able to eat well, drink lots of fluids to stay hydrated. Even if you do not gain adequately be assured that your baby is thriving.

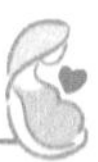

Wholesome Advice

- Healthy diet is important, but for now to help you through the tricky period of nausea, just eat as well as you can. Focus on healthy eating later.

- Check the sell-by and use-by dates on food packages to pick the freshest lot. Avoid undated meat and dairy products.

The Goodness of Folate (Folic acid)

- This vitamin prevents birth defects in a developing baby. Ideally, this vitamin should be taken 3 months before conception to ensure a healthy start and be continued for further 3 months.

- A deficiency in this nutrient causes anemia in the mother, leaving her fatigued most of the time.

Your Actions Can Impact Your Baby's Growth

Pregnancy-induced Forgetfulness

- Being forgetful about the most simple, everyday things like where you kept the keys or where you parked your car or why you called your friend, may worry you. This is normal behavior thanks to hormones, fatigue and being preoccupied with pregnancy.

Constipation

- This is a very common problem in pregnancy. Now that the muscles around the bowel are beginning to relax along with the pressure from the growing womb, your normal bowel movement gets inhibited.

- Plenty of fruit and fiber in your diet washed down with 2 liters of drinking water everyday will help. Regular exercise around the park will also help.

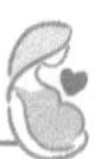

- Despite working on your fiber intake, if your constipation has not ebbed, you should consider varying your diet, cutting down on meat or dairy products whenever possible.
- Practice these alongside:
  - Massage your tummy in a clockwise direction starting from the left.
  - Take lactobacillus acidophilus supplements to increase bowel flora to break down faeces.
  - Some yoga positions safe for pregnant women may help stimulate the gastrointestinal tract – check with a qualified yoga instructor.
- Tips to ease morning sickness:
  - Eat what you feel like eating and worry less about what you should be eating.
  - Remain hydrated by drinking plenty of fluids.
  - Consume clear fluids such as water or juice diluted with water.
  - Pack in 5-6 small meals each day instead of 3 square ones.
  - Take your prenatal vitamin with a small evening meal.
  - Chill out each day; set some time aside to read a book, nap or chat with a friend.
  - Get lots of fresh air.

Common Concerns

Am I really pregnant at all?

- The fact that you do not experience many of the physical symptoms is going to worry you, but you are not the only woman to feel this way or think of this. Yours is basically a problem-free pregnancy, so enjoy.

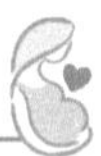

Am I going to miscarry?

* Miscarriage is most common in the first 12 weeks, but with each day and week that goes by, your pregnancy is more established. If you had some bleeding or cramping or any other concern, talk to your doctor. An ultrasound may be performed to rule out any possibility.

Nutrition

* It is hard to eat nutritiously for every meal. You may not always get the nutrients you need or in the amounts you require. Your prenatal vitamin is not a substitute for food, so don't count on it to supply you with essential vitamins and minerals. Food is important, too!

Nutrient	Food Sources
Calcium	Dairy products, dark leafy vegetables, dried beans, peas, paneer
Folic Acid	Liver, dried beans, peas, eggs, whole grain products, oranges
Iron	Fish, liver, meat, egg yolk, nuts, dried beans, peas, dried fruit
Magnesium	Dried beans, peas, cocoa, seafood, whole grain products, nuts
Vitamin B6	Whole grain foods, liver, meat
Vitamin E	Milk, eggs, meat, fish, cereals, leafy vegetables
Zinc	Seafood, meat, nuts, milk, dried beans and peas

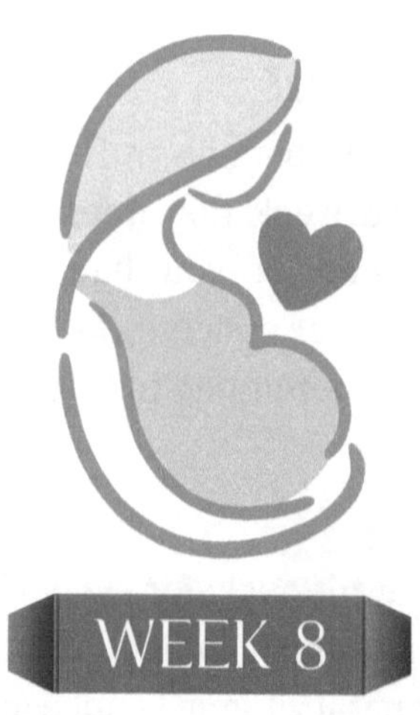

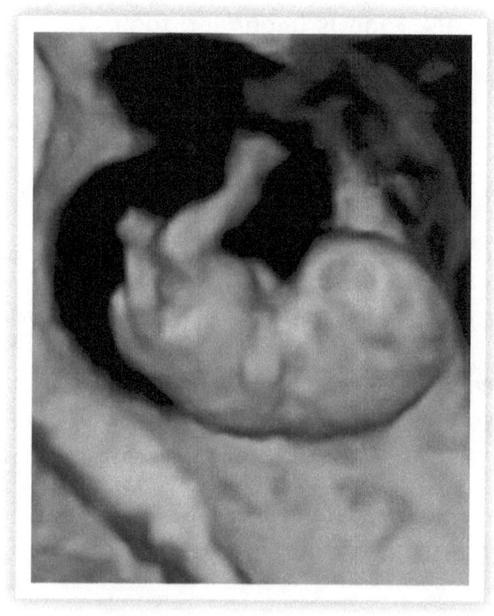

FOETUS AGE 6 WEEKS

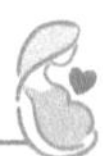

Changes in Baby

- From crown to rump, your baby measures at 1.4-2 cm or ½-¾ inch.
- From week 8, your baby graduates from being an embryo to being a fetus, literally meaning the 'little one'.
- The basics of all the vital body parts are in place now – all the main internal organs are already present.
- Baby now has the beginnings of a recognizably human face with nostrils, lips and a mouth with a tongue.
- Your baby is now covered with a thin layer of skin cells, but is still translucent.
- Baby has already started moving around inside the uterus although you are not able to feel a thing.
- Toes and fingers begin to form although they are webbed; paddle shaped foot and hand areas are clearly present.
- Initially, the arms develop faster than the legs - similarly after birth, baby will develop hand and arm control faster than leg control.
- Baby's eyelids are beginning to form and until that completes, the eyes will appear open.
- The digestive tract especially the intestines are continuing to grow.
- The dental buds have formed in each jaw - these will become baby teeth.
- Heart function is now more developed with the heart pumping about 150 beats a minute (twice the adult rate).

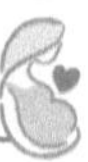

Changes in You

- The uterus is still only the size of a tennis ball.

- Hormonal changes can make you prone to mood swings and weepiness; quite similar to premenstrual tension, only longer.

- Your metabolic rate is increasing by 10-25%; your heart rate by about 10 beats per minute.

- The uterus tightens and contracts throughout pregnancy but you may not be feeling this right now.

- You may experience gastrointestinal problems such as diarrhea - it may be your body's way of quickly removing any food that isn't good for your system.

Why excessive saliva?

- One other early symptom of pregnancy is excess saliva. Sometimes your saliva tastes funny or strange that you don't find it comfortable to swallow, and sometimes the saliva glands just go into overdrive. The extreme situation is when you need to spit it out all the time though this is not a common condition. The good part is it only lasts until the first trimester, after which it diminishes.

Good to Know

Gingivitis during pregnancy

- You may wonder why I am having bleeding or sore gums after becoming pregnant. Well, many women either develop problems with gums and teeth or their condition worsens during pregnancy. Gingivitis during pregnancy hits women more often during the first trimester itself and it may worsen and continue being a problem even after delivery.

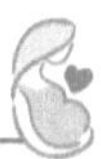

Gingivitis Causes

- It commonly occurs because of neglect. Improper brushing of teeth and infrequent flossing leads to accumulation of plaque on the teeth and this eventually irritates the gums.

- Gingivitis may develop during times of hormonal changes and that's why for some people it develops as early as puberty. Gingivitis during pregnancy, during periods and in women who are using oral contraceptive pills worsens because of the changes in hormones.

- Gingivitis can also happen to people who have poorly aligned teeth as this causes plaque to be trapped.

The developing baby

- Initially there are 3 layers of cells, all equally essential, that go on to create the different systems of the body.
- The innermost layer develops into heart, lungs, liver, thyroid gland, pancreas and bladder.
- The middle layer becomes the skeleton, muscles, sex organs, blood cells and kidneys.
- The outer layer becomes the skin, sweat glands, hair, nails and tooth enamel.

You are not the only one...

- 78% of all women experience insomnia during pregnancy, especially in the first trimester.
- 75% of women experience some form of nausea and vomiting during pregnancy at varying proportions.

Wholesome Advice

- Worry about the obvious dangers like smoking, drinking,

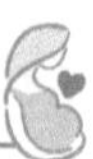

saunas and raw meat and leave the rest as they are inconclusive and debatable. For concerns such as manicures, microwaves, cell phones, computers, hair dye, eating fish, etc., approach your doctor for advice. Don't delve deeper into things and get all wired up in the process.

- Weight gain in excess of 35 pounds (15.89 kgs) makes you prone to gestational diabetes and high blood pressure - talk to your doctor if you are concerned. The average woman gains 30 pounds (13.62 kgs) during a normal pregnancy; she should gain a little more if she was underweight to begin with and a little less if she was overweight.

- Treat yourself to one piece of chocolate or sweet every day unless you have diabetes or some medical condition where it is just not viable to do this. But if you are well, a treat like this is good for your system.

Your Actions Can Impact Your Baby's Growth

Hormonal stress

- It is comforting to know that emotional stress does not seem to have a definite negative impact on pregnancy - the growing baby is very strong and resilient.

- However, stress does have its effects: the quickening heart rate or elevation of stress hormones.

- How you deal with stress is of key relevance; you have to keep your pregnancy in perspective and work on strategies to reduce anxiety instead of making wrong choices and indulging in unhealthy habits. Stress easers include:

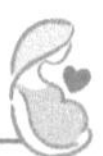

- Understand and accept that your feelings are normal.
- Trust your emotions and have confidence in yourself.
- Keep sharing and talking about your feelings with your partner or a friend.
- Do your best but always take care of yourself first.
- Educate yourself on what is happening with your body and keep yourself posted on what to expect ahead.
- Release your energy through safe exercises like walking, swimming, etc.
- Join a yoga class.
- Give yourself an occasional treat such as a chocolate or ice cream.
- Listen to soothing music or read an inspiring book.
- Time spent alone is good but too much can be depressing, especially if it is not well-occupied; chat with friends, surf the net, read the papers or watch TV.
- Consider counseling if you cannot shake off pregnancy blues.

What if I ate junk food yesterday?

- Don't punish yourself over this - you are not as perfect as you would like to be. Just do your best to eat a balanced, healthy meal as much as possible, drink plenty of water and don't forget your prenatal vitamins. For any concerns/changes you are not too comfortable with, consult your doctor for advice.

Should I avoid caffeine totally?

- Caffeine found in tea, coffee, carbonated drinks and chocolate can have a harmful effect on the digestive system and prevent the absorption of iron. Cut down to one cup a day or cut it out totally if you can.

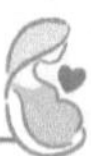

What should I eat?

- It is important to eat a variety of foods to ensure you get your nutrients. Foods are the best sources of nutrients because unlike vitamin and mineral supplements, food derived nutrients deliver nutrients in a natural balance. If you know the basics and were eating healthy before you became pregnant simply add an extra:
  - 300-500 calories of nutritious foods daily
  - 25 gm of protein
  - 800 mg of calcium
  - 0.4 mg of folic acid
  - 40 mg of iron

What if I wish to color my hair?

- It is advisable to dye your hair the original color. Pregnancy hormones may alter the hair texture causing your hair to respond differently to coloring agents. Although it is safe to dye your hair, you may not get the desired results.

Nutrition

- Dairy products are important to you during your pregnancy as they contain calcium and also vitamin D which aids in calcium absorption. Calcium helps keep your bones healthy, and your baby needs it to develop strong bones and teeth.

- During pregnancy you need at least 1200mg - 1500mg of calcium a day. That is equivalent to 3-4 glasses of skimmed milk. Calcium also helps prevent high blood pressure and may lower your risk of developing preeclampsia (high blood pressure and a large amount of protein in the urine).

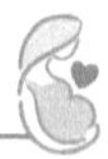

- In addition, your body stores calcium in the latter part of pregnancy to draw from, during breastfeeding.

- Milk, yoghurt, cheese and ice cream are good sources of calcium. Other foods include broccoli, spinach, salmon, sardines, chickpeas, sesame seeds, almonds, cooked dried beans, and tofu. Some available foods are now calcium fortified such as orange juice, breads, cereals and grains.

- If you plan to keep you calorie intake in check, choose low fat dairy products. Some choices include skimmed milk, low fat yoghurt, cheese and ice-cream. Calcium content remains unaffected in low fat dairy products.

- You can increase the amount of calcium in your diet in other ways. Add powdered non-fat milk to soups. Make fruit shakes with fresh fruit and milk. Cook rice and oats in skimmed or low-fat milk. Some foods interfere with calcium absorption such as tea and coffee.

- For the lactose intolerant, you can still get your calcium from other sources outlined above. Some dairy products you may choose and their serving sizes outlined below:
    - Cottage cheese (Paneer) - ¾ cup
    - Hard cheese - 30 grams
    - Custard or pudding - 1 cup
    - Milk - 225 grams
    - Natural cheese - 40 grams
    - Yoghurt - 1 cup

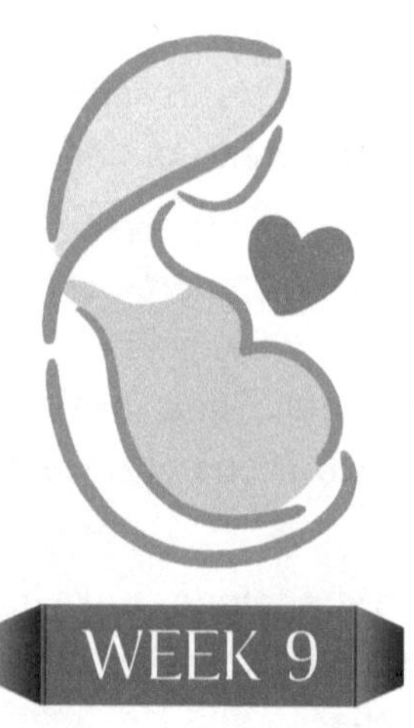

WEEK 9

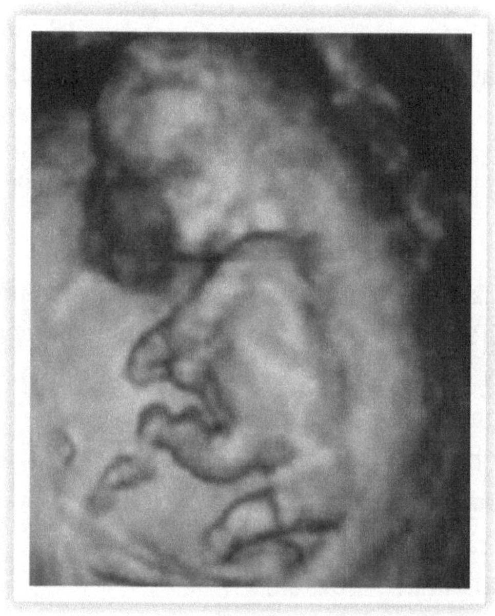

FOETUS AGE 7 WEEKS

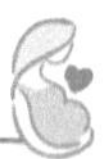

Changes in Baby

- From crown to rump, your baby measures at 2.2-3 cm or 1-1¼ inch, the size of a medium green olive.

- This week, your baby is looking less like a tadpole and more human - the tail at the bottom is shrinking and disappearing and the face is more rounded.

- Hands and feet continue to form along with the fingers, toes and elbows.

- Internal organs such as testes and ovaries start to develop this week, but the external genitals don't have noticeable male or female characteristics yet.

- The eyelids almost cover the eyes now, the intestines are growing longer and the pancreas, bile ducts, gall bladder and anus have formed.

Changes in You

- As your uterus grows larger your waistline starts to thicken as well.

- The hCG levels are at their peak this week. This week is going to probably be rough, but starting next week things start to get better as your hormone levels stabilize.

- For most women, the side effects of the first trimester still continue to bother, especially the nausea and vomiting - expect this to last the entire month. It almost always subsides by the end of next month.

- Changes in body shape and function may affect you, causing you to feel less attractive in general, especially if this is your first pregnancy.

- Your second prenatal visit is around the corner - it will be briefer this time. Pelvic exam is not required unless something is amiss.

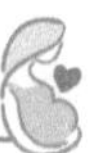

Good to Know

If you can't handle dairy products?

- If milk leaves you with a lot of gas, you are probably lactose intolerant; in your case milk does little good to your body. Lactose intolerance happens when there is an inadequate supply of the enzyme lactase, required to digest milk sugar - lactose. Symptoms include:
  - Gassiness
  - Bloating
  - Indigestion
  - Cramping ranging from mild to severely uncomfortable
  - Diarrhea

Metallic taste

- Many women experience a metallic taste in their mouth. Though unpleasant, it is not unusual and is most likely to fade away in the second trimester along with most of the other discomforts.

- Chewing ice may help.

Discharge

- Increased vaginal discharge is yet another annoying but normal surprise of pregnancy.

- You will need to use pads for the discharge caused by increased hormones and blood flow to the skin and muscles of the vagina area.

Gestational times - some facts...

- In general, the larger the animal the longer the pregnancy - for human beings it is 40 weeks. The average gestational time for some other mammals:

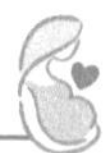

- Elephant - 95 weeks
- Sea lion - 52 weeks
- Whale - 52 weeks
- Horse - 47 weeks

Wholesome Advice

- Exercise has its benefits. During the first trimester, you should let your body guide you and do what feels right. Don't feel bad if you are not able to even go for walks because of your overwhelming fatigue or extreme queasiness. You can exercise later when you feel better.

The Do's and Don'ts of Pregnancy Exercise

Do's

- If you feel light-headed or breathless, stop immediately
- Try and rest in-between workouts
- Drink plenty of fluids and have proper meals to stay hydrated and energized. Pregnancy and exercise increases the need of both, you and your baby
- Dress appropriately and exercise in cool atmospheres to prevent overheating
- When getting up from a lying down position, roll unto your side first and then onto all fours
- Ten minutes warming up and ten minutes cooling down are essential

Don'ts

- Avoid any form of exercise or activity that can cause abdominal trauma
- Don't raise both legs at any time
- Unless your abdominal muscles are strong do not engage in single leg raises as well
- Avoid standing in one spot for prolonged periods
- Do not push yourself till you are totally exhausted

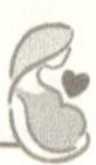

- Avoid engaging in exercises that could tip your balance
- Do not perform exercises on your back after the middle of the second trimester
- Do not exercise if you have a temperature

Your Actions Can Impact Your Baby's Growth

Eating for two!

- Research has proven that you need only an additional 300 calories per day during pregnancy, which roughly means an apple and a glass of milk!

- Smaller meals of 5-6 servings per day ensure your blood sugar levels remain stable and your digestive system isn't burdened.

- Add this with 8 glasses of water and your system stays hydrated while your metabolism stays right.

Using the computer

- According to research, extended use of computer during pregnancy is nothing to worry about. If at all, pay attention to your posture to avoid backache and keep your feet raised using a foot support.

First trimester fatigue

- Your fatigue is a by-product of all the work your body is doing at present. Your brain is receiving less oxygen, your blood pressure is lower now, you are growing a whole new organ for your baby (the placenta) and your sweat glands right to your kidneys are working doubly hard. Lastly, extra weight caused by fluid retention means more weight to carry around.

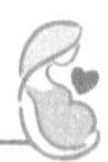

Common Concerns

What are the pros and cons of sharing my pregnancy news now?

- You receive a lot of attention and maybe even gifts; you also get to share the excitement with many others

- You have the excuse of showing odd behavior or attitude such as mood swings or wanting to rest at a gathering full of people and get away with it

- Your can benefit from other peoples experiences and receive wholesome advice

- Your pregnancy seems to last forever

- The only thing anyone ever asks you is 'when are you due?' or, 'is it a boy or a girl?'

- If you have a miscarriage or other problem typically occurring in the first trimester, everybody gets to know about it

What are the pros and cons of waiting to share the news until later?

- You and your partner have the time to adjust and plan

- If you miscarry or have other problems, you can deal with it privately

- You won't have to suffer unsolicited comments or advice from various sources

- You may have to lie or come with excuses to deal with your pregnancy discomforts e.g. lie to disguise your need to lie down

- You may have to deal with an interrupted social life

- You cannot use the excuse of pregnancy to avoid unpleasant tasks

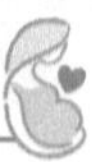

- You are going to hurt some people since you didn't tell them sooner

Nutrition

- Fruits and vegetables are important during pregnancy. You can add a variety to your diet because they are seasonal.

- They are an excellent source of vitamins, minerals and fiber. You get your supply of iron, folic acid, calcium and vitamin C from them.

  Tasty low-cal sources of vitamin C:
  - Strawberries - 1 cup contains 94mg of vitamin C
  - Orange juice – 1 cup contains 82mg of vitamin C
  - Kiwi fruit – 1 medium contains 74mg of vitamin C
  - Broccoli – ½ cup cooked contains 58mg of vitamin C
  - Red peppers – ¼ of a medium contains 57mg of vitamin C

- Vitamin C can be very important during pregnancy. It is important for fetal tissue development and iron absorption. Some studies indicate that vitamin C helps prevent preeclampsia. Deficiencies have been linked to premature births. It helps build the amniotic sac. The recommended daily dose is 85mg. Besides your prenatal vitamin, you can depend on fruits and vegetables for your daily dose. Every day try to eat one or two servings of fruit high in vitamin C and at least one dark green or deep yellow vegetable for extra iron, fiber and folic acid. Fruits and vegetables you may choose and their servings outlined below:
  - Grapes - ¼ cup

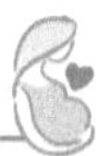

- Banana, orange, apple - 1 medium
- Dried fruit - ¼ cup
- Broccoli, carrots and other veggies - ½ cup
- Potato - 1 medium
- Leafy green vegetable - 1 cup
- Vegetable juice - ¾ cup

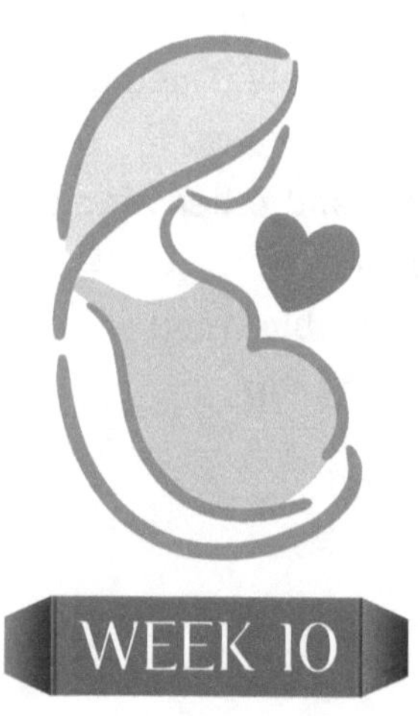

WEEK 10

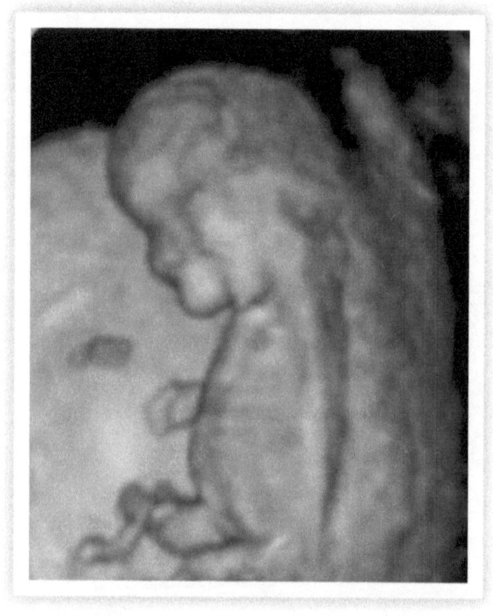

FOETUS AGE 8 WEEKS

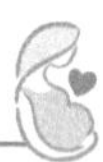

Changes in Baby

- From crown to rump, your baby measures at 3.1-4.2cm or 1 ¼ - 1 ¾ inch, the size and shape of a medium shrimp.

- The prenatal test, CVS is usually conducted between this week to week 12.

- Now that the baby is starting to put on weight, your baby's weight is close to 5g or 0.18 oz.

- Most congenital malformations occur during the embryonic period - it is encouraging to know that a critical phase is safely behind you.

- Although few malformations occur during the fetal period, it pays to stay away from drugs and other harmful exposures throughout your pregnancy as fetal cells can be destroyed at any time during pregnancy.

- By week 10, all of your baby's vital organs have formed.

- The tail has disappeared totally and the fingers and toes are no longer webbed.

- The skeleton bones are starting to form; the eyes now look closed since the lids are more developed.

- Rapid brain development is taking place with almost 2,50,000 neurons being produced every minute!

- With a boy baby, testosterone is now being produced by the testes.

Changes in You

- You still may not show much, though your uterus is the size of a large orange.

- Though the majority of women rely on the basic clues to determine pregnancy in the first trimester, sometimes

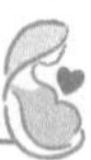

you may notice a slight staining around the time you would normally expect your periods; this is called implantation bleeding.

- Implantation bleeding is caused by a shedding of uterine cells when the fertilized blastocyst first burrows into the womb. You may experience tender breast or mild cramps akin to period symptoms.

Good to Know

Couvade Syndrome

- 80% of expectant fathers experience the Couvade syndrome, which is psychosomatic in nature; they gain weight, lose sleep, have cravings and morning sickness along with their partners. This condition is believed to be caused by empathy, guilt or anxiety.

Your eyes

- Now, your body retains extra fluid. Because of this, the outer layer of your eye or cornea thickens by about 3%.
- This change starts around now and lasts till about 6 weeks after the delivery.
- At the same time, the pressure of fluid within your eyes decreases by 10%.
- These two events may cause you to have a slightly blurred vision - you may find hard contact lenses in particular difficult to wear. Your eyes will normalize after you give birth.

Myths and misconceptions about twins

- Twins usually skip a generation
- Fraternal twins are always a boy and a girl

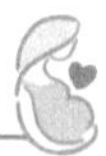

- Twins with 2 placentas must be fraternal twins
- You have to buy 2 of everything for your twins
- All twins must be born by cesarean section
- Identical twins always look exactly alike
- It is impossible to breastfeed twins
- You must have taken fertility drugs if you have twins

Wholesome Advice

Thyroid conditions and the pregnant woman

- During the first half of pregnancy, a pregnant body's need for the thyroid hormone called thyroxin increases. Thyroid problems can either take the form of hypothyroidism (when there is a lack of the hormone) or hyperthyroidism (when the gland is overactive). 1 in 50 women experience hormone deficiency or hypothyroidism during pregnancy.

- Wash your hands thoroughly throughout the day if you have not started doing so. After using the washroom or handling raw meat, it becomes especially important, since this simple activity can help prevent the spread of many bacteria and viruses.

- If you still feel the nausea, here is a trick you can try. Soak cucumber in water for 10 minutes and then give them a try. This may just work for you.

Your Actions Can Impact Your Baby's Growth

The Caffeine Buzz

- Medical research shows that caffeine in moderation does not harm the mother or the fetus. Moderation equals to 300 mg of caffeinated beverage in a day! Of course it is best to eliminate caffeine altogether during your pregnant months, but low levels are found to be safe.

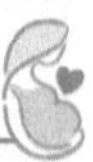

Drink	Amount	Caffeine level
Brewed coffee	8 oz (~235 ml)	100 – 300 mg
Instant coffee	8 oz (~235 ml)	50-190mg
Espresso/cappuccino	8 oz (~235 ml)	40-70mg
Decaf coffee	8 oz (~235 ml)	1-8mg
Brewed black tea	8 oz (~235 ml)	35-175mg
Green tea	8 oz (~235 ml)	8-30mg
Iced tea	12 oz (~355 ml)	65-75mg
Soft drink	12 oz (~355 ml)	30-60mg
Hot cocoa	8 oz (~235 ml)	3-30mg
Chocolate milk	8 oz (~235 ml)	2-7mg

Alcohol and pregnancy

- Alcohol and pregnancy just don't gel! It causes your heart rate and that of your baby's to drop. This may lead to reduced circulation and deprive baby of important nutrients and oxygen. So remember when you drink, so does your unborn baby. Exposure to alcohol leads to various physical abnormalities, mental retardation and fetal alcohol syndrome or FAS. No amount of alcohol is safe during pregnancy - that goes for beer, wine, cooler, liquor and mixed drinks.

- FAS is a form of mental retardation that has characteristic physical deformities. It can lead to behavior and learning problems in the baby. FAS is preventable - the safest thing you can do is to not consume any alcohol during pregnancy.

Risk of Smoking

- It is a proven science that cigarette smoke reaches the fetus. From the mother's blood stream, these toxins travel through the placenta and enter the unborn baby's circulation. The poisons constrict the blood vessels

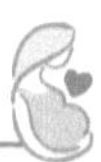

thereby preventing baby from receiving vital nutrients which are important for its growth and development.

- It is just not good for baby to be around polluted air. Smoking can cause miscarriage, stillbirth, low birth weight or sudden infant death syndrome (SIDS). A baby born to a smoking mother has a greater chance of being born small, underdeveloped and sickly. Baby may be born early before her lungs mature and may have difficulty breathing. Tobacco in other forms such as cigars, snuff or pipe tobacco is harmful as well.

Common Concerns

I am expecting twins. How much extra nutrition do I need?

- In a gist, more than when you are carrying a singleton. You will need to consume more calories, more protein, more vitamins, more calcium and more iron. Each day you will need an additional 250 calories, 25 gm of protein, 20 gm of iron supplement and a higher dose of folic acid as determined by your doctor.

Should I worry about sex since I am carrying twins?

- Because women carrying multiples have an increased chance of delivering prematurely and since orgasms can stimulate uterine contractions, conventional wisdom advises these women to abstain from orgasm during the final trimester. Studies recently suggest that there is no correlation between intercourse and premature delivery of twins.

Is it true that I will put on a lot more weight with twins?

- You are more likely to gain extra weight with multiple

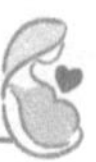

fetuses. For a normal-weight woman, a weight gain of 35 to 45 pounds or 15.75 - 20.25 kg for a twin birth is recommended. However, some women do not gain as much due to the added stress on their bodies.

What is the average length of pregnancy with more than one baby?

* Delivery of twins is pushed until about 37th week of pregnancy and triplets until about 35th week.

Nutrition

* Protein supplies you with amino acids which are critical for the growth and repair of the embryo/fetus, placenta, uterus and breasts.

* Pregnancy increases your protein needs.

* Try to consume 6 oz (~170 gm) of protein each day during the first trimester and 8 oz (~225 gm) a day in the next two trimesters.

* Protein should however make only about 15% of your total calorie intake.

* Many protein sources are high in fat. If you need to watch your calories, look out for low fat protein sources. Some protein foods you may choose and their serving portions are outlined below:

  - Chickpeas (Kabuli channa) - 1 cup
  - Cheese, mozzarella - 1 oz (~28 gm)
  - Chicken roasted, skinless - ½ breast
  - Eggs - 1
  - Milk - 8 oz (~235 ml)
  - Peanut butter - 2 tablespoons
  - Yoghurt - 8 oz (~225 gm)

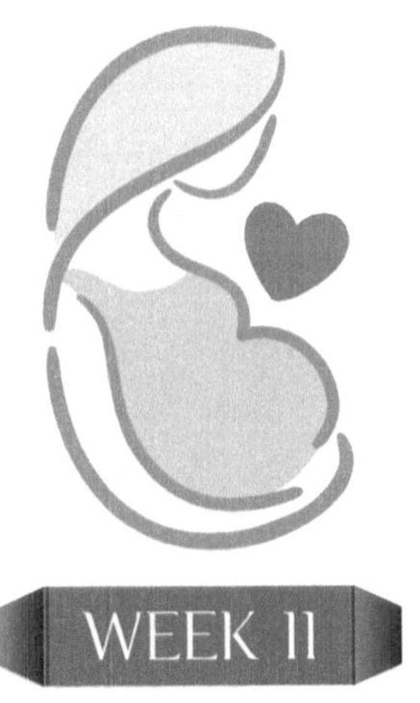

WEEK 11

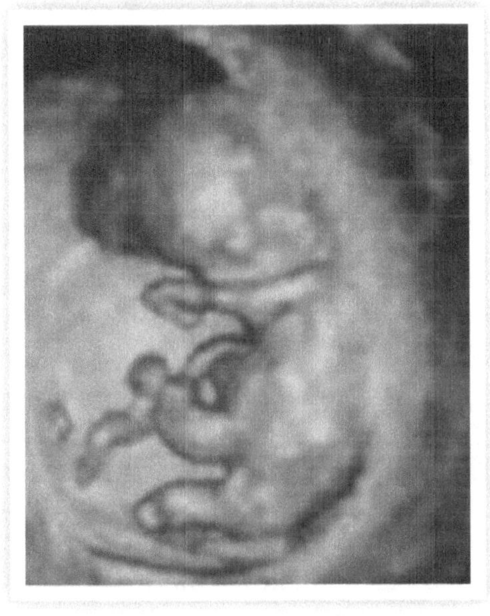

FOETUS AGE 9 WEEKS

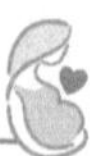

Changes in Baby

- From crown to rump, your baby measures at 4.4-6 cm or 1 ½ - 2 ½ inch, the size and shape of a peanut. Fetus now weighs about 0.3 oz (8gm).

- Week 11 begins the time of rapid growth; starting now, right up till the mid-point of pregnancy or the 20th week, your baby will increase 30 fold and triple in length.

- Blood vessels in the placenta are multiplying to keep up with the nutrients supply to the fetus.

- External genitalia are starting to show obvious differences although it won't be until 3 weeks later when the gender features are more complete.

Changes in You

- The first trimester is almost over - your uterus now is big enough to fill your pelvis and you can feel it in your lower abdomen.

- For some women pregnancy brings about changes in their appearance i.e. either an increase in hair and nail growth or hair loss.

- Some have glowing skin while others suffer an acne breakout.

- These changes have been attributed to hormones, increased blood volume or a phase in the growth cycle of hair and nails. Whatever the reason these changes are not permanent.

Vaccinations in pregnancy

- Some vaccines are safe to have while pregnant and some are not. The general rule is to avoid live vaccines while

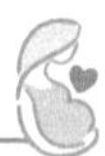

pregnant. Live vaccines contain the virus which can be transmitted to the fetus via the placenta and prove harmful to the fetus. In principle, you must postpone plans to conceive for at least 3 months after being vaccinated.

- It is preferred that all vaccination be carried out prior to pregnancy. Vaccinations in pregnancy are most harmful in the first trimester. Some vaccines are considered 'safe' during pregnancy because they are made out of inactive or killed viruses and can be given if the mother has chronic illness or is at high risk because of lifestyle.

Good to Know

Placenta tidbit

- In the next week or so, the placenta will start functioning. The placenta is also called the 'afterbirth' because after the baby is born, the mother delivers the placenta. It is an organ that exists only during pregnancy, and after your baby is born, your body will expel it. While the placenta can filter out infections and some other harmful materials, it cannot dispose chemicals such as caffeine, alcohol, cocaine and cigarette by-products. A mother's stress hormones can also cross the placenta to her baby.

Your baby now!

- Your baby has plenty of new tricks. The baby can open its mouth and close its fist. It can suck its thumb. Not amazing enough? Consider this: your baby is barely the size of your thumb and it is sucking its thumb now!

- Most mothers get to hear their baby's heart beat for the first time at around 10 - 12 weeks of pregnancy, or at the 2nd prenatal visit. Baby's heart beats typically about

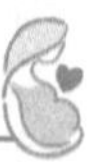

120-160 beats per minute while most mothers' pulse averages at 70-80 beats per minute!

Wholesome Advice

- *Pee emergencies:* Never go anywhere without using the bathroom before you leave even if you just went, look for a bathroom once you arrive at your destination, and carry plenty of tissues in case you need to do 'it' on the roads (sometimes you just can't hold on).

- You have nothing to worry about when it comes to bathing, except for the temperature. In general, avoid hot tubs or baths that raise your temperature above 102 or 103 degrees Fahrenheit or 39 degrees Celsius.

- If increased hormone is causing your skin to break out, cleanse your skin more and increase your intake of fresh fruit, vegetables and water.

- Lean forward when you pee to empty your bladder fully and reduce the number of times you have to visit the washroom. Do not try and cut back on water since you may need more, not less fluids during pregnancy.

Your Actions Can Impact Your Baby's Growth

Leg cramps

- These are quite common during pregnancy and can be quite uncomfortable. They are not dangerous. There are several theories as to why leg cramps happen.

  One, your leg muscles are tired from carrying the extra weight of pregnancy. That is why the starting point is almost always from the 2nd trimester and only gets worse as you grow heavier.

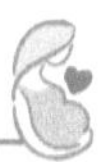

Two, the blood circulation in your lower extremities are not optimal and so the increasing weight and pressure of the pregnant uterus worsens the ache.

Finally, there is the theory about your body lacking in minerals such as calcium, magnesium and potassium. Studies indicate that this lack may lead to muscle cramping and spasm.

Things you can do to relieve leg cramps

- When you get the cramp, try straightening your leg and gently flex your foot and toes.
- Always point your toes up and not downward as this can trigger a cramp.
- Massage your calf with long strokes toward the foot.
- Apply a heat pad on the affected area.
- Avoid standing for long periods.
- Never sit cross legged as this worsens circulation.
- Walking helps.
- Rotate your ankles clockwise and then anti-clockwise.
- Drink lots of fluids.
- Load your diet with calcium rich foods viz. milk, yogurt, cheese and leafy vegetables.
- Eat a banana every day.
- Check with your doctor on calcium / magnesium supplements

Previous abortion

- If you are concerned about whether a previous abortion will now affect your ability to give birth, don't be.

- One or more abortions in the past which were free of complications and performed in a medically modern facility and in an adequate manner, poses no greater risk

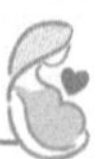

of fertility problems, ectopic pregnancy, premature birth, low birth weight, deformities or miscarriage comparatively.

* If you did have complications after an abortion such as infection or perforation, make sure your doctor is aware of the details so that you receive proper attention now.

Common Concerns

How can drinking fluid help me?

* Many women suffer from headaches, uterine cramping and other problems during pregnancy. They find that drinking more fluids helps to resolve these problems along with preventing bladder infections. Drink about 8 glasses or 1.9 liters of liquid every day. Water is of course the best form to choose. When urine is light yellow, you are getting enough water and when it is dark yellow, you need to up the fluid level.

If I exercise, do I need to eat more?

* Your nutrition needs increase during pregnancy and since you do burn extra calories during exercise, you should consume enough calories to ensure a balanced diet. A woman of normal weight before pregnancy needs to eat about 300 extra calories.

I seem to have terrible mood swings - is this normal?

* Elevated hormones can trigger mood swings. You may also find yourself fatigued more than usual which is also normal. It is all hormonal, but on your part you can take things easy and take a break if any situation becomes unbearable.

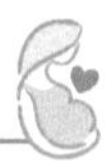

<u>Bleeding in early pregnancy and what it can mean...</u>

- Your hormone level may not be high enough to subdue your periods.

- The spotting is often a sign of implantation i.e. the fertilized egg attaching to the lining of uterus. Usually it lasts for a day or two.

- Having sex is usually not a problem, but occasional spotting may result from intercourse; refrain from sex for the time being.

- Bleeding can start and stop on its own; if the bleeding is slight and stops on its own, your chances of delivering a healthy baby are great.

Nutrition

- Carbohydrate foods provide primary source of energy for your developing baby.

- These foods ensure that your body uses protein efficiently.

- Foods from this group are almost interchangeable, so it should be easy to get all the servings you need.

- Some carbohydrate foods you may choose and their serving sizes are outlined as follows:

  - Cereal or rice, cooked - ½ cup

  - Cereal, ready to eat or instant - ~30 grams

  - Bagel - ½ small

  - Chapati - 1 large

  - Bread - 1 slice

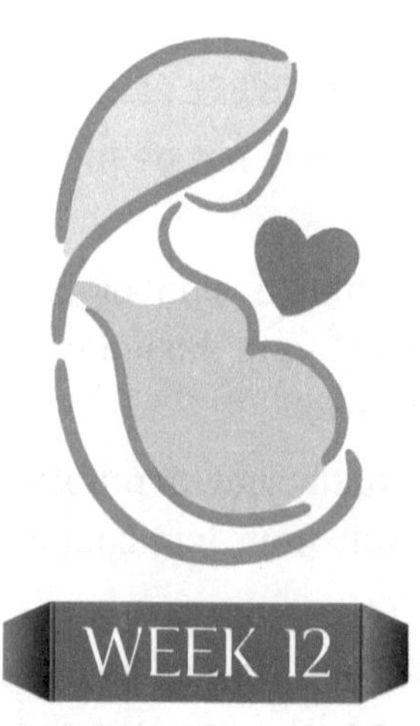

WEEK 12

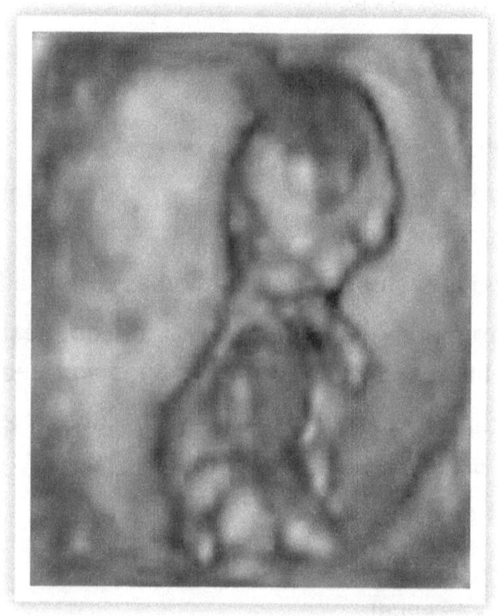

FOETUS AGE 10 WEEKS

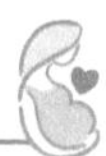

Changes in Baby

- From crown to rump, your baby measures at 6 cm or 2½ inch, and weighs about ½ oz or 14 grams. Fetus is the size of a plum.

- The end of 12th week marks the end of the first trimester. The baby is quite active at this stage but you cannot feel the kicks and stretches yet.

- Baby is already swallowing little amounts of amniotic fluid.

- Baby also passes urine which constitutes the amniotic fluid.

- Baby has wrists, ankles, tiny fingers and toe nails - baby is able to make a fist.

- Baby's head is quite large in proportion to the rest of its body.

Changes in You

- Key hormones are now being produced by the placenta - your risk of miscarriage drops significantly.

- You may develop a hormone-related dark line on your abdomen called linea nigra which will fade after baby's birth.

- By this stage, you may have put on about 10% of your total pregnancy weight. Conversely you may have lost weight if you had morning sickness.

- The urge to urinate frequently may start now as well, If not already started.

- Bleeding gums are again due to hormonal changes - avoid brushing too vigorously.

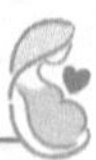

- You will find yourself worrying less about miscarriage, but now your screening tests occupy your mind a lot. Discuss the options and the pros and cons with your doctor.

- Up to the 12th week of pregnancy, your uterus fits inside your pelvis. By the end of the month, your uterus will have expanded up out of your pelvic cavity so the pressure on your bladder will ease up.

Good to Know

Amniotic fluid

- Your baby floats in amniotic fluid, which was formed by the placenta and your baby's own urine. Right now, the fluid level is at ~100 ml and the fluid level will be highest around week 34, averaging at ~800 ml.

Breast issue

- The most rapid breast gain occurs in the first trimester and the last trimester with a break in between. Generally the breast weight gain for most women is 1-2 pounds (450-900g) or one to two cup sizes. Some women get a lot bigger, 2 or more cup sizes and some don't at all.

Umbilical cord

- Now that baby's hands are well developed, she is able to use the cord as her first plaything; she will reach out and grasp it often.

Blood vessels

- An average woman has 9 pints of blood; on the average a pregnant woman adds 1.8 pints during pregnancy. Much of the excess blood is lost during childbirth.

- Your entire circulatory system increases its capacity after a week into pregnancy.

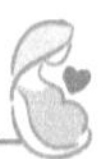

- The entire first trimester your body works to fill the extra room in your blood vessels and priority is given to providing blood to the developing placenta, nourishing the baby and removing waste.

Wholesome Advice

Pregnancy bleeding - An overview

- Roughly 1 out of 4 women will experience vaginal bleeding during their pregnancies; it is particularly common, but doesn't necessarily mean that there is a problem. Many blood vessels are being formed with the growth of the placenta that an occasional tiny vessel breaks and you start to spot or bleed a little. A good way to tell if the pregnancy is safe is by the amount of pain associated with the bleeding. A small amount of painless vaginal bleeding doesn't amount to much, but should the bleeding be heavy, accompanied with cramps and backache you should contact your doctor right away. That is to say slight bleeding in early pregnancy which is painless, brief and the blood is red or pinkish with no fragments of tissue is non worrisome.

- If you feel your uterus is big and pants are tightening, make sure you don't forget to buckle your seatbelt when in a vehicle. Your uterus now holds the baby, placenta and amniotic fluid.

Your Actions Can Impact Your Baby's Growth

- Dizziness when you stand up or sit too quickly will result in not enough oxygen to go around especially to your brain. Be easy when you stand or sit.

- Urinate when you feel the urge. Your kidneys are working

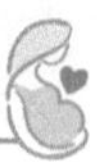

harder now to filter increased blood and make extra urine to flush out waste.

Common Concerns

Can an ultrasound be able to tell at this stage if I am having a boy or a girl?

- It will almost be too early to tell if it is a boy or a girl. The purpose of scanning right now is to date the pregnancy accurately, to check if you are carrying a single baby or more, to check the heartbeat of baby and maybe to look at the nuchal fold. It is illegal to know the unborn baby's gender and your doctor too will not divulge it to you.

Can my baby sense the outside world?

- Your baby is beginning to respond to the world outside the uterus. If you try to press your abdomen your baby may respond by moving away.

How does my baby change during the first trimester?

- This trimester is one of greatest change period – your baby grows from a collection of cells, the size of a head of a pin to a fetus the size of a softball. Organs begin developing and your baby begins to look more normal, all in the first 13 weeks.

Nutrition

- Some women think they can eat all they want just to increase their calories. Don't fall into this trap. It is unhealthy for you and your baby if you gain too much weight during pregnancy, especially in the first trimester.

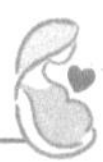

Carrying and delivering your baby becomes tough and shedding those excess pounds post pregnancy becomes an ordeal. Once the baby is out, most of you will want to return to 'normal' clothes at the earliest, so don't let those extra kilos interfere with your goal.

Junk food

- Now that you are pregnant, break the habit of junking if you love junk food and skipping your first meal of the day, the breakfast. Your dietary habits affect your unborn child as well. Proper nutrition takes some planning on your part but it can be done. It is easy to have a quick fast food bite, but think about the harm you are doing to your baby. Avoid foods that contain a lot of fat and sugar. If you work, take healthy foods with you for your lunches and snacks. Stay away from fast food and junk food no matter how tempting.

Late night snacking

- Late night nutritious snacks are beneficial for some women. However, snacking at night is unnecessary. Food in your stomach late at night is no good if you suffer from heartburn, indigestion or nausea.

Fats and sweets

- Unless you are underweight, you may want to be cautious with fats and sweets. Many of these foods are high in calories and low in value. Eat them sparingly. Instead of munching on potato chips, reach for an apple, cheese slice or peanut butter and bread. You will satisfy you hunger without compromising on nutritional value. Some

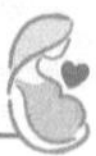

fats and sweets you may choose and their serving sizes are as follows:

- Sugar or honey - 1 tablespoon
- Oil - 1 tablespoon
- Jam or jelly - 1 tablespoon
- Salad dressing - 1 tablespoon
- Butter or margarine - ½ teaspoon or less

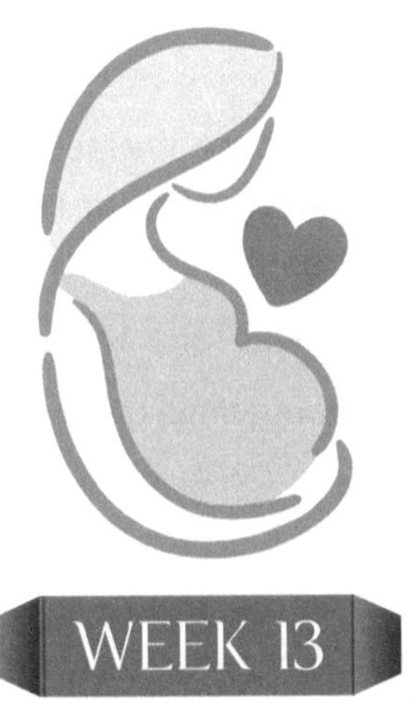

WEEK 13

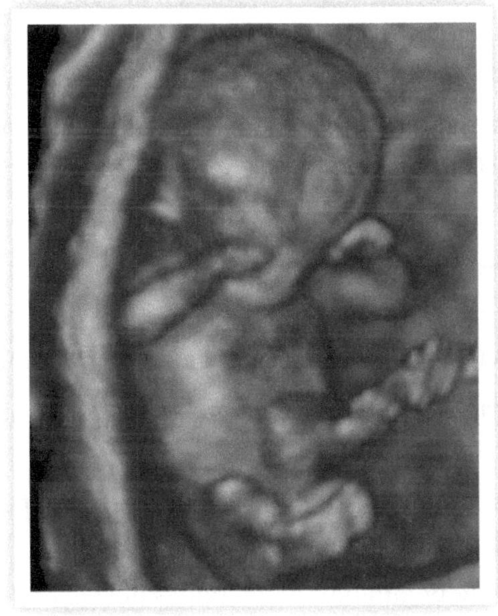

FOETUS AGE 11 WEEKS

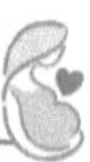

Changes in Baby

- From crown to rump, your baby measures at 6½ - 7.8 cm or 2½ - 3 inches, and weighs about 1 oz or 20 g. Fetus is the size of a medium goldfish.

- Baby's vocal cords will form this week.

- Baby is also hiccupping now; this helps strengthen baby's diaphragm and prepare its respiratory system for breathing.

- Kidneys can make urine and its bone marrow is making white blood cells, necessary for fighting infection after baby's birth.

- As you enter the 2nd trimester, all of your baby's organs, nerves and muscles are formed and just beginning to function together.

- Baby's eyelids are fused together and will not reopen until week 30 to protect the developing eyes.

Changes in You

- You will start to feel less sick and more energized as the days pass - in 2-3 weeks you could be free from nausea.

- For some women, the aversions to taste and smell sticks on till the end of pregnancy.

- You are probably starting to show your pregnancy - time to wear loose fitting clothes.

- Shoes are beginning to feel tight - now is a good time to invest in shoes that accommodate your widening feet.

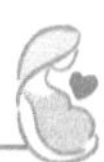

Good to Know

Uterus tidbit

- For 38 weeks of pregnancy, your uterus is your baby's home. It starts out the shape and size of a pear and then grows until it reaches the bottom of your ribcage. It is a 3-layered organ: the outer layer is made of connective tissue, an inner layer comprising of about four sub-layers of smooth muscle & elastic tissue and a lining which when you are not pregnant is shed every month.

- During pregnancy, your bowels are moved around and displaced so much by your uterus that your appendix ends up just beneath your diaphragm instead of in its normal place deep within the pelvis.

Wholesome Advice

Second trimester scan

- Also known as anomaly scan, most women are offered second trimester scan between weeks 18 - 22 to check on the baby's development. Second trimester scan is detailed and the whole scan can last for nearly half an hour.

- Don't worry yourself sick about your baby if you are under constant nausea attack. If you are able to swallow your prenatal vitamin, water and some form of food, you and your baby are probably fine. At this point your baby is still too small and its caloric needs are not that great anyway. Knowledge means power, but if you get too much of it you will end up worrying about a lot of things. Know when and where to draw a line.

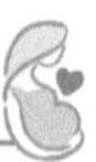

Your Actions Can Impact Your Baby's Growth
Urinary Tract Infections (UTIs)

- During the 1st trimester your urinary tract is working overtime to filter waste from your blood - this means frequent trips to the washroom. Don't be tempted to cut down on water because of this inconvenience because your body and baby need to get rid of waste to grow.

- Pregnant women are at a higher risk for UTIs due to the softening or the urethra because of hormonal changes.

- UTIs in pregnancy are more likely to develop into kidney infections which can in turn increase the odds of pre-term delivery.

- A woman is more likely to get UTI if she has had them in the past. Some women, more than others are more vulnerable to infection.

- Typical symptom is the feeling of having a constantly full bladder but not able to pass much fluid when in the bathroom; pain, a burning sensation when you urinate; bloody, cloudy or foul smelling urine; lower back or abdominal pain; a low fever. Sometimes the symptoms don't show.

- It is important to treat UTI right away to prevent kidney infections.

Ways to prevent UTIs

- Wipe from front to back to keep bacteria out of the urethral area.

- Wear cotton underwear; avoid synthetic materials and thongs.

- Avoid skin irritants such as perfumed toilet napkins or soaps.

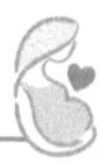

- Urinate frequently or whenever you get the urge to prevent urine from standing still in the bladder.

- Avoid caffeine for now as it is an irritant to the urinary tract.

The Flu Shot

- This is a safe vaccine made of inactive viruses and egg whites.

- This shot is recommended to pregnant women during the flu season.

- Pregnant women with chronic ailments such as asthma or diabetes are advised to go for this shot since flu becomes dangerous for them.

- Flu shot protects again the serious strains of flu but not the familiar infections like the common cold.

Exercise basics during pregnancy

- If your doctor has okayed your decision to exercise, you should be aware of some basics before starting on your regime. Exercise basics apply more now than ever as your body is different from the pre-pregnancy days. For instance, your heart rate and blood pressure rise faster at the start of the activity when you are pregnant than when you were not pregnant. Therefore, well-planned warm up and cool down sessions are important for anyone who works out, but becomes all the more essential for the pregnant exerciser because demands of pregnancy are different. Ask your doctor for advice.

Common Concerns

Can a deficiency in nutrients cause a miscarriage?

- There is no concrete evidence suggesting a link between

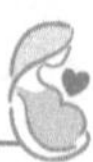

lack of a certain nutrient or even moderate amounts of all nutrients to miscarriages. Please follow the diet advised by your doctor.

Nutrition

• Caffeine is a central nervous system stimulant found in many beverages and foods including tea, coffee, cola drinks and chocolates. Caffeine is also found in headache medicines.

• Research shows that you may be more sensitive to caffeine during pregnancy comparatively. High caffeine intake has been associated with low birth weight babies and a smaller head size in newborns. Some researchers have gone as far as to say that caffeine use leads to miscarriages, stillbirths and premature labor.

• Cut down on caffeine or better still eliminate it from your diet. Too many negative associations i.e. it crosses to your placenta to the baby, it can affect yours and your baby's calcium absorption.

• Increased intake can lead to breathing problems in your newborn; if you are jittery, your baby may suffer from the same effects.

• Read labels on over-the-counter medications for caffeine. Up to 2 cups (not mugs) of regular coffee or its equivalent is probably permissible as that is less than 200mg a day. Still it is a good idea to stop consuming caffeine altogether to have a healthier you and a healthy baby.

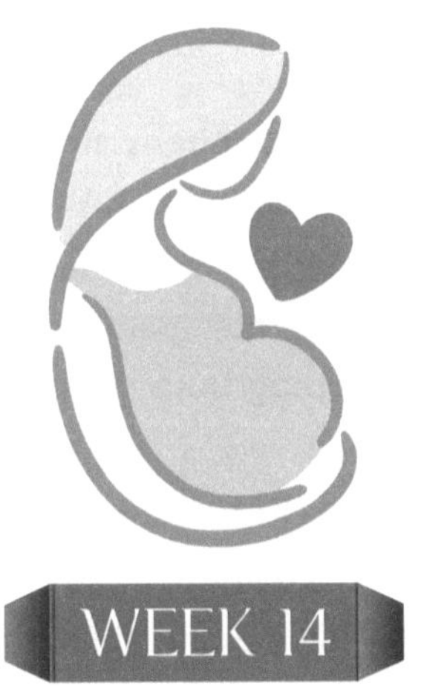

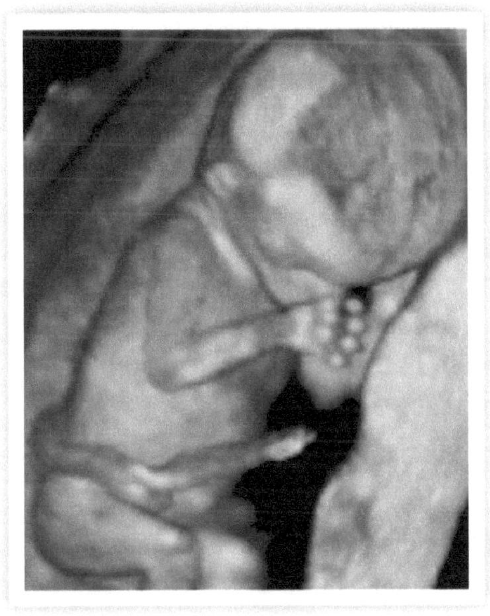

FOETUS AGE 12 WEEKS

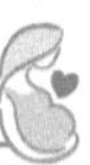

Changes in Baby

- From crown to rump, your baby measures at 7.8 – 10.1 cm or 3-4 inches, and weighs about 1oz or 20g.
- The reproductive site has the most action this week - for a boy baby the prostate gland is developing and the ovaries are descending from the abdomen to the pelvis for the girl baby.
- Thyroid gland begins its function by producing hormones.
- Your baby's skin is very thin; head hair and eyebrows are growing and may have pigment if baby has the genes for dark hair.
- Bone marrow has begun to produce blood cells which was previously produced by the yolk sac.
- Your baby rarely sits still; it is either yawning, stretching and hiccupping or wiggling its toes and fingers but none of these movements can be sensed by you.

Changes in You

- Regardless of breast size, they may have already started to produce colostrums or pre-milk, an antibody-rich fluid that feeds baby and keeps it healthy for the first few days of life.
- The amount of amniotic fluid increases by quite a bit this week.
- Many of the discomforts such as moodiness, exhaustion, etc. are easing up but they tend to linger until the baby is born.
- If fatigue is bothering you this week, make sure it is not due to lack of iron - apart from your iron supplement, try to get your extra iron from food sources as this mineral is better absorbed through food.

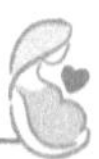

- Plenty of food cravings and aversions are starting to hound you now - give in to cravings, but in moderation.

Good to Know

- If you are eating spicy foods now, your baby may just grow up liking them too.

- Many women miscarry more than once in their lives; about 1 in 36 women will have 2 miscarriages due to mere chance. Having a miscarriage does not affect the woman's ability to carry a baby to term in the future.

- During pregnancy your waistline may increase by up to 20 inches to accommodate your growing baby.

- Human Chorionic Gonadotropin (hCG) is a hormone unique to pregnancy, as it can only be produced in the placental cells. It enters the circulatory system and is traceable in the woman's urine after a few days of conception.

Baby's Senses

- Your unborn child is growing physically, mentally and physiologically, with all the five senses developing during those months in the uterus. While still in the womb, the unborn baby with all its organs in place; will breathe, move, swallow amniotic fluid, react to stimuli and prepare itself for life outside the womb. The learning and conditioning that happens in the nine months are crucial.

Wholesome Advice

Looking great during pregnancy

- When you are pregnant, you need to feel nurtured. Set yourself a routine which should be practiced daily in the

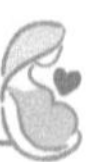

mornings and evenings. That way you will also stay in touch with your body throughout your pregnancy term and in turn help motivate yourself towards regaining your pre-pregnancy form after delivery.

- Don't hesitate to request your boss for a more flexible work schedule.

Your Actions Can Impact Your Baby's Growth

Help for varicose veins

- Varicose veins are merely blood vessels engorged with blood. Though not dangerous or harmful to mother and baby, they are unsightly and do cause discomfort to the mother, especially in the lower extremities and pelvis.

- Your body has got more blood and fluid now and that means the veins have more blood and fluid to drain. Pregnancy hormones cause the muscle lining and valves to relax causing the veins to work harder.

- Excess weight and pressure of the uterus compound matters further.

- Plus, when you stand for longer periods, blood in your lower body will take a longer time to reach your heart and lungs because baby, placenta and uterus act like a big road block.

- Some women are more predisposed to varicose veins because of their family genes.

- Keep off your feet. Avoid standing too long and sit with your feet elevated as often as possible. Use a footstool wherever necessary to take the pressure off the back of your legs.

- Uncross your legs. Do not cross your legs; this reduces circulation.

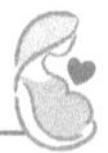

- Wear maternity support stockings to give your legs some support. Use suitable shoes with good arch support.

- Exercise and stretch regularly. Gentle stretching of your body can help blood to return to your heart so it doesn't collect in your veins.

- Get off your feet as much as possible by reclining on either your left or right side but not flat on your back.

Common Concerns

Why is pregnancy making me so tired?

- Throughout pregnancy, more so in the first trimester, your body is working hard. During this time your body is making the placenta and your hormone levels and metabolism are going through changes; your blood sugar and blood pressure is lower. Combined, all these factors contribute to make you feel tired.

Am I likely to feel nauseous throughout my pregnancy?

- Nausea can last for a few weeks to a few months. For most women, the nausea subsides after the third month although mild nausea lingers on throughout pregnancy. It is often triggered by certain smells and this again varies from one woman to another.

Can exercising increase the risk of miscarriage?

- In low-risk pregnancies, exercising does not increase the chance of miscarriage. However, if you have any condition or fall into the high-risk category, you must seek medical advice before exercising.

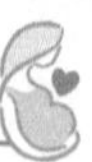

When does bone development in a fetus take place?

- In the 6th week fetus has gained a complete skeleton which is not yet made of bone. It is fashioned of cartilage; the true bone cells replace the cartilage between days 46-48. The appearance of the bone cells marks the end of the embryonic period and the beginning of the fetus stage. Although by 12 weeks, joints and bones are all formed, the ossification or bone hardening takes much longer.

Nutrition

- Being overweight at the start of pregnancy may present special problems. You may be advised to gain less weight than the average 25-35 pounds required for a normal-weight woman.

- You will probably have to choose low-calorie, lower-fat foods to eat. A visit to the nutritionist may be necessary to help you develop a healthful food plan. You will be advised not to diet during your pregnancy.

- Extra weight brings in more problems, including gestational diabetes or high blood pressure; backaches, varicose veins and fatigue intensify for heavier women.

- If you put on much during your pregnancy, beyond what your doctor advised, chances of a Cesarean delivery increases.

- If you are overweight, visits to your doctor will be more often. Ultrasounds may be needed to help establish your due date because it is harder to establish the position and size of the fetus.

- Extra layers of abdominal fat may make manual

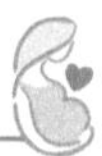

examination harder. Your doctor may order for gestational diabetes tests, along with other diagnostic tests as you near your due date.

Iron myth

- Certain foods e.g. spinach, egg yolk; though rich in iron, cannot be absorbed through the intestines. Most nutritionally important is the 'elemental (pure) iron' which means the amount of iron available for absorption. It is best to begin on iron supplements early in pregnancy or before if possible in order to store extra iron. Your doctor will prescribe the appropriate iron supplement when required.

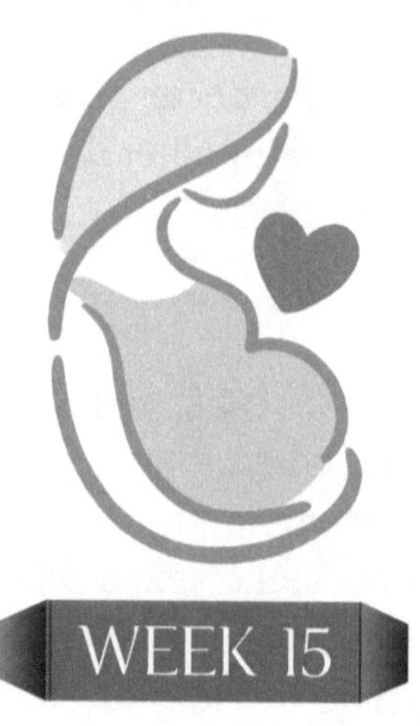

WEEK 15

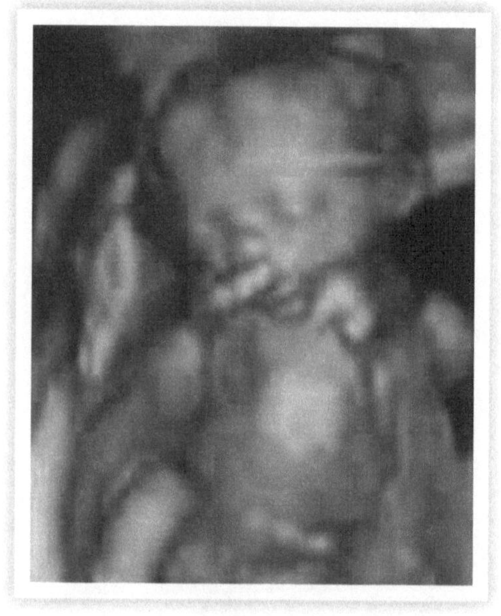

FOETUS AGE 13 WEEKS

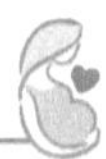

Changes in Baby

- From crown to rump, your baby measures at 4 inches, and weighs about 1¾ oz (~50g).
- Baby's body is now growing faster than the head.
- All of baby's tiny organs, muscles and nerves are beginning to function.
- Baby's facial muscles are flexing and developing.
- The liver has begun to secrete bile; the pancreas has begun its production of insulin; the bone and marrow, part of the skeletal system, continue developing.
- Bones that have already formed are hardening now, which increases your need for calcium.
- Fine colorless hair called lanugo (a Latin word for wool) starts to develop - most of this hair will shed before the birth.
- Skin is very transparent that you can see the blood vessels through it.
- By the end of this week your baby will be able to form a fist.

Changes in You

- Your womb is now starting to show and grow out of your pelvis - the bump is more noticeable.
- Your milk glands may be preparing to begin production.
- Skin changes such as spider veins and darkening of moles and freckles can be expected.
- You may begin to feel Braxton Hicks contractions (false labor) - you may feel it more after a round of exercise.
- You are still emotionally vulnerable and find yourself easily annoyed than in your pre-pregnancy days.

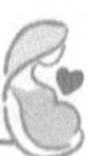

- Hormone release by your placenta, ovaries, adrenal glands and pituitary gland continue to surge this week and will continue to do so throughout your pregnancy.

- Right now, the extra blood is mostly plasma, the fluid part of blood. During the first 20 weeks, your body produces more plasma, more quickly than red blood cells.

Why nosebleeds & nasal congestion

- Nose problems are common, particularly in the colder months of the year. They can be uncomfortable, but fortunately don't last long nor do they present serious repercussions. The membranes inside your nose may either dry out, bleed easily or become swollen. As a result you may experience nasal stuffiness or nose bleeds quite frequently.

What causes it?

- The membrane lining the nasal cavity may dry up.
- This lining has a tendency to swell up because of the increased blood flow during pregnancy.
- Circulation changes, caused by changes in hormones during pregnancy can cause the nasal membranes to act up.

Good To Know

Blood pressure

- During the first 24 weeks of pregnancy your systolic blood pressure or the top number will drop by 5 to 10 points and your diastolic pressure or the bottom number will drop by 10-15 points. After that they will gradually return to pre-pregnancy levels.

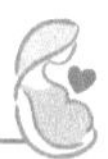

Food additives during pregnancy

- Just what are food additives during pregnancy and does it affect you or your baby during pregnancy is a concern with many pregnant women. Additives are substances added to food because of processing, packaging and storage. Additives are also added to flavor, enhance flavors, color and preserve food's freshness. Most food additives are safe during pregnancy unless you are allergic to them. From what is known so far, there is a very remote chance for the developing fetus to suffer from any side effects owing to chemical additives in food.

Your Lungs now

- Since baby takes up more room now, there is less space for your lungs to expand. Pregnant women have to breathe faster to compensate for this change and to meet the increased oxygen demands of both the mother and the fetus. Coupled with that, the hormone progesterone will also give you the feeling that you are not getting enough air.

Wholesome Advice

- Most doctors can spend only 15 minutes with you max, so be prepared with a list of questions relevant to the stage of your pregnancy. The good thing about prenatal visits is that you will have more than 10 sessions during your entire pregnancy, which gives you ample opportunities to discuss your concerns.

OTC or Over the Counter Medication

- There are a lot of drugs which were once safe to buy off the shelf but are now best avoided. As a pregnant lady, it

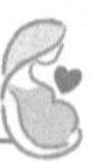

is advisable to follow your doctor's advice on what you should take. Always inform the pharmacist or doctor about your pregnancy, especially in the early months when you may not be showing.

The Plain Facts

* Some drugs can cause an early miscarriage

* Drugs are thought to account for 2-3 % of birth defects

* Very few medications are completely safe

Teeth Care

* Your teeth need attention too. Keep up with dental appointments - have your teeth professionally cleaned by the dentist at least once during your pregnancy to prevent gum disease and infections.

* Brush your teeth and tongue at least twice a day. Keep up with the flossing. Be gentle as your gums are softer than before and will bleed more easily.

* Chew sugarless gum after meals if you do not get a chance to brush.

* Don't miss your prenatal vitamins and calcium supplements as directed by your doctor to help strengthen your teeth and keep your mouth healthy.

* Fluoride is important for the development of baby's teeth. You do not need to depend on supplement if you drink or cook with fluoridated tap water (bottled water does not usually contain fluoride).

* You can get your fluoride supply from tea brewed in fluoridated water, fish with edible bones, kale, spinach, apples and non-fat milk.

* Avoid sugary foods as much as possible, another reason

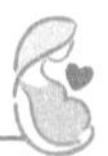

to not indulge in too many chocolates and pastries, biscuits and fizzy drinks.

Iron deficiency

- If you do not get the required amounts of iron to allow your body to produce more red blood cells, you may become anemic.

- Anemia is a result of insufficient red blood cells in your blood and therefore not enough protein hemoglobin is able to transport oxygen to various tissues of your body.

- You become more susceptible to illnesses and you tire easily.

- Despite this your baby gets enough iron even if you don't.

I am in my second trimester and don't have any health issues. When is the safest time to fly?

- Now is the best time to travel. Long flights in the first trimester increase the risk of bleeding and having a miscarriage. Long flights in the final trimester would be dangerous for both mother and baby. Hence, the middle (second) trimester with adequate care is the safest time.

My vision is blurry although I had a recent prescription done. Should I get a new refraction done and new glasses or contact lenses?

- Swelling during pregnancy is not restricted to ankles and hands but everywhere else including the cornea. Swelling of the cornea can cause a temporary miscalculation for your prescription eyeglasses. Your eyes should revert to normalcy after you have your baby.

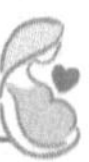

Common Concerns

What causes hypotension (low blood pressure) during pregnancy?

- There are two kinds: supine hypotension and postural hypotension. The first type is caused by the enlarging uterus putting pressure on large blood vessels such as aorta and vena cava. This happens when you lie down and can be prevented by not sleeping or lying on your back. The second type is caused when you rise rapidly from a sitting, kneeling or squatting position. Gravity causes blood to leave your brain which causes a drop in blood pressure. Avoid this by rising slowly.

Eating out during pregnancy

- Eating out during pregnancy is the main concern with many pregnant women. While you are concerned about eating right, you are also inclined to want to let go a bit. Eating out during pregnancy also depends on the trimester you are in because your moods and taste buds will determine the food choice and how much of it you can eat. With a little planning, you can obtain the necessary nutrients when you eat out.

Nutrition

- You will probably start to need an extra 300 calories to your meals to meet the needs of your growing baby and your changing body.

Eating eggs during pregnancy

- Eggs impart several key nutrients in the form of protein, fats, minerals (such as zinc and selenium) and vitamins A,

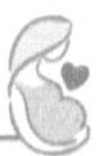

D and some B vitamins, which make it a necessary food item during pregnancy. An egg during pregnancy is undoubtedly one of the most nutritious foods and is healthy for the pregnant woman but safety should not be overlooked.

Milk, cheese and cream during pregnancy

- Milk, cheese and cream are dairy items that are healthy to eat during pregnancy as they provide the much needed and easily absorbed calcium (essential for your baby's bones and teeth), protein and some vitamins. Dairy foods are also a good source of protein for women who are on a meat-less diet.

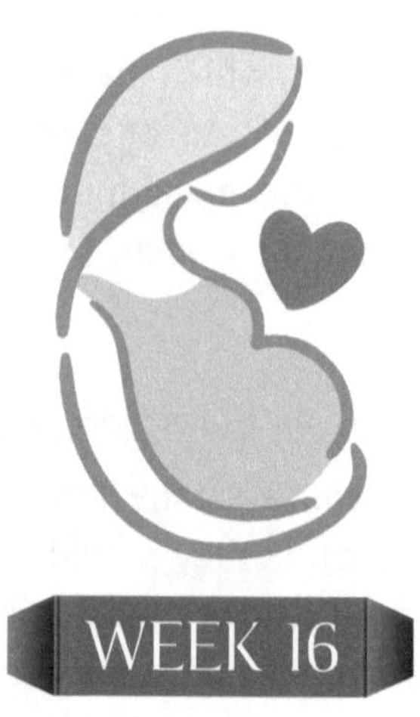

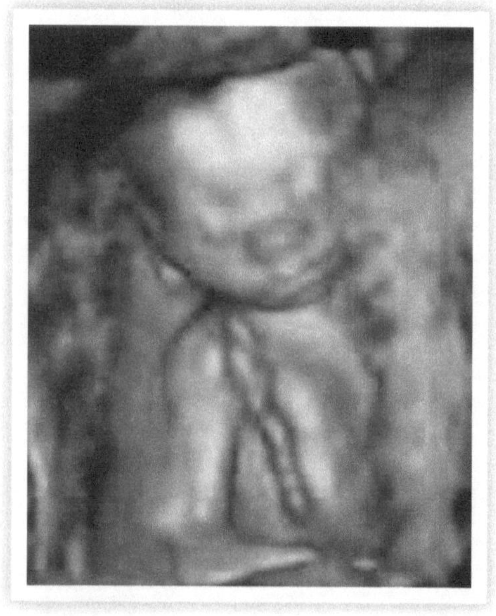

FOETUS AGE 14 WEEKS

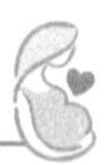

Changes in Baby

- From crown to rump, your baby measures at 4-5 inches, and weighs about 3 oz or 80 gm. At this point, baby can fit in the palm of your hand.

- With a girl baby, millions of eggs are forming in her ovaries this week.

- Starting now, baby's eyes are sensitive to light.

- Baby's hiccups are becoming common although these cannot be felt at all - since her trachea is filled with fluid and not air, the hiccups do not produce the typical sound.

- Your baby can now swallow, hiccup, kick and swim.

- Eyebrows, eye lashes and fine hair begin to appear.

Changes in You

- It is time to invest in looser outfits now as your clothes start to feel tighter.

- Your kidneys are processing 25% more blood than usual.

- Your uterus is getting about 5 times more blood as compared to the pre-pregnancy stage.

- Extra blood and mucous will make you more prone to nasal congestion.

- You may notice you are breathing slightly faster this month; you may also be having shortness of breath.

- Your uterus is higher and more forward and this is altering your center of gravity.

- Your navel is starting to protrude - this is because of the pressure from your growing uterus.

- There is about 250 ml of amniotic fluid around your baby, about a cupful.

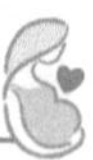

- Heat rashes are more common because of the damp skin. Pregnant women perspire more because of the hormones and the heat being produced by the developing baby.

Good to Know

Miscellaneous

- By this week, your baby's taste buds resemble a mature adult's.

- When taking calcium supplements, it is best to take smaller amounts a couple of times a day to allow for the best absorption.

Twin type

- Twins are two offspring produced by the same pregnancy. Twins can be either monozygotic ("identical"), meaning that they develop from one zygote, which splits and forms two embryos, or dizygotic ("fraternal"), meaning that they develop from two different eggs. In fraternal twins, each twin is fertilized by its own sperm cell.

Wholesome Advice

Calcium supplements

- When looking for a calcium supplement, read the label carefully. Ideally, the label will list how much elemental calcium is available in each tablet. If elemental calcium is not stated the following data can help you figure out.

- Elemental calcium accounts for these percentages of the following compounds: Calcium Carbonate - 40% ; Calcium Citrate - 21%; Calcium Lactate - 13%; Calcium Gluconate - 9%.

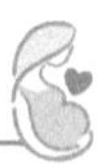

- Supplements that contain calcium citrate can be taken on its own without food while calcium carbonate has to be taken with food for optimal absorption.

- Many antacids contain calcium carbonate which is a more convenient and affordable way to ingest your calcium.

- Avoid the natural source calcium pills such as those produced from oyster shell or bone meal as they may contain lead or other toxic metals.

- If you are taking both calcium supplement and iron supplement, be sure to take them at different times of the day. Each mineral will be better absorbed on its own.

Your Actions Can Impact Your Baby's Growth

Ways to reduce swelling

- *Keep off your feet:* Avoid standing for long periods; keep your feet elevated at work so to prevent the pressure at the back of your legs.

- *Warm baths:* Baths in warm water help to compress your tissues and reduce swelling.

- *Eat more protein foods:* Increase in protein will increase the protein pressure of your blood and draw the fluid from your tissue back into your bloodstream.

- *Lie down:* Lying on your side can help your body to reabsorb extra fluid by taking pressure off the main veins.

- *Swimming:* A great form of exercise for pregnant women, and the water pressure helps with your circulatory system.

- *Natural diuretics:* These include watermelon, parsley, coriander and cucumber. Natural fluid reducers help the body excrete excess fluid.

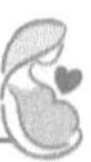

Common Concerns

Do all babies develop at the same rate in the womb?

- All babies grow at about the same rate until 12 weeks. After that, there are a lot of changes proving that every baby is unique. Your baby's growth and size at birth depends on genes, whether he is your first baby or not, whether there are maternal factors at play, your diet and lifestyle.

If all my baby's organs are already formed do I still need to be careful about avoiding certain foods?

- Keep to the same food regime as before: wash all fruits, salad ingredients and vegetables well, avoid raw and undercooked meat and unpasteurized dairy products as there are potential dangers to your baby even in the latest weeks of pregnancy.

Can problems with my blood sugar cause dizziness?

- Pregnancy affects blood sugar; either high blood sugar (hyperglycemia) or low blood sugar (hypoglycemia) can make you feel dizzy or faint. Pregnant women are routinely checked for problems with blood sugar.

What can I do if I have a problem with blood sugar?

- You can avoid the problem or improve it by eating a balanced diet; do not skip meals and go for a long time without eating. If you need help, see a dietician and if your test shows diabetes, your doctor will be able to guide you further.

Radiation and pregnancy

- Radiation comes in many forms. Ionizing radiation emitted from x-rays can be worrisome to many pregnant

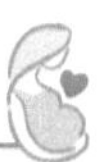

women, and rightfully so. It is dangerous for the developing fetus to be exposed to high levels of ionizing radiation. Steps should be taken to avoid or reduce the danger during pregnancy since it is something we can voluntarily prevent. Radiation exposure to the fetus can result in miscarriage and severe birth defects.

Nutrition

- Pregnant women should snack more, more so during the second half of pregnancy.

- You should have 3 to 4 snacks a day in addition to your regular meals. There are a couple of catches though.

- Firstly, snacks must be nutritious.

- Secondly, your meals must be smaller and only then snacking makes sense.

- Your goal should be eating enough, so important nutrients are always available for your body's use and for use to your growing fetus.

- Quick and easy snacks are preferable, especially now.

- Planning and effort will be necessary to make your snacks healthy and easily available. Preparation in advance is the key.

- Cut fresh vegetables for later use in salads and for munching with low-cal dips. Peanut butter, popcorn (low salt / sugar variety) are good choices.

- Low fat cheese, yoghurt is another one to go for. Fruit juices and fresh cut fruits are good and refreshing. If fruit juice is high in sugar, cut down on the sugar by adding water.

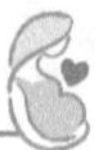

Salt and swelling

- Excess salt is not to be blamed for the swelling pregnant woman's face. Don't restrict your salt intake unless advised by your doctor. Salt does cause your body to retain fluid but your fluid requirements will double up to support the increase in blood volume and to replenish the amniotic sac. So don't ignore the craving for salt as it is nature's way of ensuring your body gets some. Choose iodized salt over sea salt.

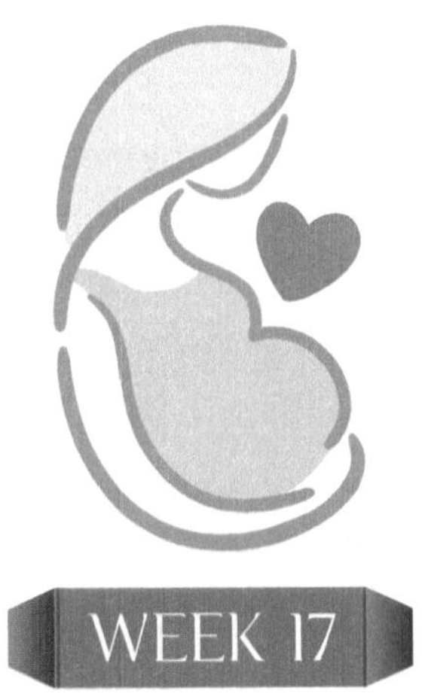

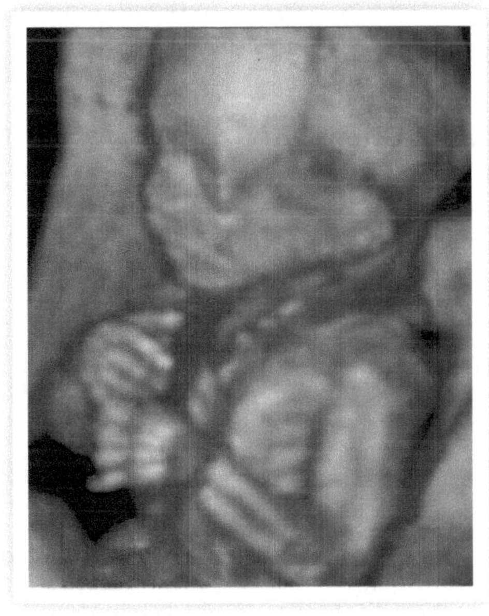

FOETUS AGE 15 WEEKS

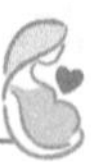

Changes in Baby

- From crown to rump, your baby measures about 5-6 inches and weighs about 100 gm.

- The fetus is the size of your palm spread wide open.

- While still big, the head is beginning to look in proportion with the rest of the baby's body.

- Incredible changes are happening now; fat is beginning to form this week and will continue in the weeks that follow. Known as adipose tissue, fat helps to keep baby warm and gives the baby energy.

- Baby's small heart is pumping 24 liters of blood a day.

- Your baby can now hear sounds outside your body and may even be startled by it.

Changes in You

- You are showing your pregnancy more now.

- Your uterus is about 2 inches (4-5cm) below your belly button.

- Maternity clothing is a must for comfort sake.

- The rest of your body is changing as well - a gain of 5 - 10 pound or 2.5 - 3.5 kg is normal.

- The uterus now fills the pelvis and starts to grow into the abdomen.

- Though your uterus doesn't float around, it is not attached to one spot either.

- If you have had a previous pregnancy, you may feel your baby's first movements.

- The urge to pee frequently should have passed by now.

- Expect to be more absentminded and forgetful now, but

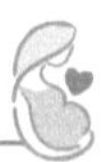

according to research there is no link between pregnancy and your memory.

White and odorless vaginal discharge

- The combined effect of hormones progesterone and oestrogen, causes your vagina to secrete more mucus than before. This discharge, termed leucorrhea comes in greater quantity now that you are pregnant. Discharge is composed of vaginal and cervical fluids, old cells shed from the vaginal walls and normal fungus and bacteria (vaginal flora).

- You will notice this increase from around week 18 or even earlier.

- The secretion should be clear, milky white and odorless.

- It should not itch or cause any pain.

- Its function is to keep your vagina area moist.

- There can be lots of it and is likely to increase as your pregnancy progresses.

Good to Know

Ultrasound

- Ultrasound tells us about baby's anatomy; it reveals the different structures in the brain and the heart.

- Fluid can be evaluated to make sure there is sufficient quantity.

- Placental details can be assessed.

- Baby's growth can be monitored through ultrasounds in high risk pregnancies. Despite all the important information, ultrasound cannot determine or detect chromosomal or other abnormality invisible to the eye.

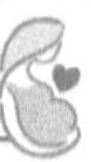

Leg cramps

- Don't stand for long periods

- Rest on your side whenever you can.

- Using a heating pad on the affected area helps but do not use it longer than 15 minutes at a time.

- Potassium helps in reducing leg cramps; sources include raisins and bananas. Add this mineral to your diet before leg cramps get to you.

Wholesome Advice

Music

- Now that baby's sense of hearing is developing, it's a good idea to introduce her to your favorite tunes. It would be a good idea to play soothing music which your child can hear later on in the house or car.

Sodium

- During pregnancy, keep your sodium under 3g or 3000mg a day.

- Too much sodium causes water retention, swelling and high BP which can become a problem for you.

Your Actions Can Impact Your Baby's Growth

Round ligament pain

- Round ligaments are attached to each side of the upper uterus and to the pelvic side wall.

- During pregnancy these ligaments are stretched and pulled and as such become longer and thicker.

- Your movements can stretch and pull these ligaments causing pain and discomfort called round ligament pain.

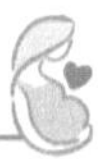

- It is indicative of a growing uterus.

- The pain is on one side or both sides, or it may be worse on one side than the other.

- The pain is not harmful to you or your baby in any way; it is just an uncomfortable feeling to bear with.

- Lying down and resting will make you feel better.

- Talk to your doctor if pain is unbearable or if any other symptoms arise such as vaginal bleeding, fluid loss from the vagina or severe pain.

Common Concerns

Colds and flu during pregnancy

- Interestingly, colds and flu during pregnancy will not hurt your baby, unless your temperature shoots up to 102°F and above. The worse can happen if you fall really ill in the first trimester. In the later stages, if you become dehydrated, the risk of premature labor increases. Pregnancy is surely the worst time to feel so miserable, but what makes it even harder is the fact that you cannot be taking over-the-counter medications as you used to before.

Is sex harmful to baby?

- Your baby is adequately protected by amniotic fluid. When you have an orgasm, your uterus contracts and hardens as it usually does at other times. Avoid sex if you have a history of miscarriages or premature labors, or bleeding.

Non-ionizing radiation and pregnancy

- Non-ionizing radiation that emanates from common household appliances and gadgets causes no harm to

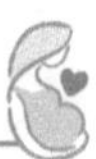

your pregnancy. Still, many pregnant women are troubled when they use microwaves, cell phones, electric blankets or when they watch TV. There is no way to avoid non-ionizing radiation which is emitted from almost every home or office machine you use these days.

Nutrition

- Whether a vegetarian diet is ideal during pregnancy is an important question especially for vegetarians. It can be, if you watch closely the types and combinations of foods you eat.

- Since meat is eliminated from vegetarian diet, you have to ensure sufficient calories are consumed to meet your energy needs.

- Calories need to be the right kind, derived from appropriate sources such as fresh fruits and vegetables.

- Empty calories have to be avoided since they have little or zero nutritional value to it.

- Your goal is to eat sufficient protein to provide energy for the fetus and you.

- By eating a wide variety of whole grains, dried beans and peas, dried fruits and wheat germ, you will be providing your body with iron, zinc and other trace minerals required.

- You must find other sources of calcium, and vitamins B2, B12 and D. Seek your doctor's advice on supplements.

Healthy soy (soybean)

- If you are pregnant and vegetarian, soybean becomes all the more important because of the protein in it. The

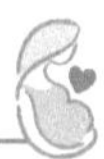

popular belief that protein is best obtained from animal products is a myth. When pregnant, your need for protein increases because you are replenishing your own body, alongside you are providing your baby with the raw materials for its growth. Soy is a plant food that is a 'complete' protein and contains all nine of the essential amino acids.

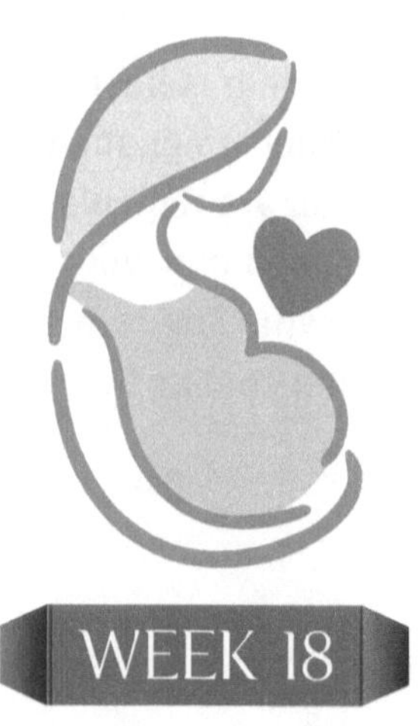

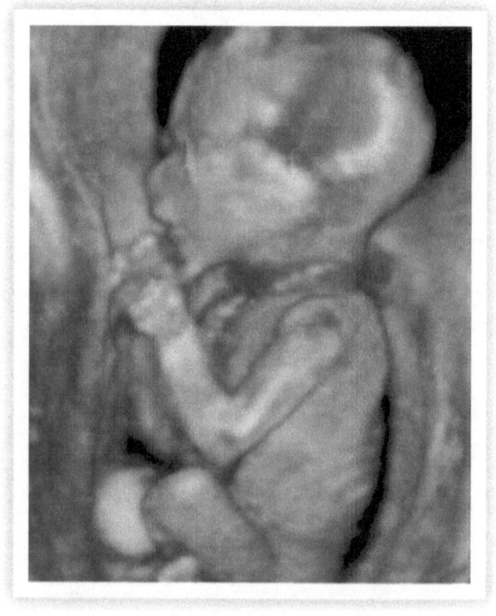

FOETUS AGE 16 WEEKS

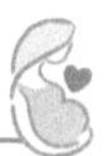

Changes in Baby

- From crown to rump, your baby measures at 5-5 ½ inches, and weighs slightly above 140 gm.

- Your baby continues to have hiccups which you cannot hear, but can probably feel, especially if this isn't your first baby.

- Brown fat has begun to form under baby's skin - this acts as an insulator after birth when baby adapts to change from the uterus to the outside world.

- A good dose of amniotic fluid is being swallowed every day by the fetus; interestingly, some scientists believe this act keeps the amniotic fluid at the appropriate level constantly.

- This week, the bones of the ear form completely along with the part of the brain that processes signals from the ears — therefore at this stage, baby is able to hear your heart beating, your stomach rumbling or movement of blood through the cord.

Changes in You

- During this week and the coming weeks, the first fetal movements can be felt.

- You may experience aches and pains in your legs, tail bone and other muscles.

- By 18 weeks into your pregnancy, your placenta is more than an inch thick; it contains thousands of blood vessels which carry oxygen and nutrients to your baby.

- Your skin may go through a color change - it will darken around the nipples, navel, armpits, inner thighs and perineum.

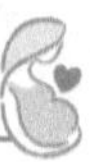

Itch and skin rash during pregnancy

- Your growing abdomen may contribute to the skin becoming stretched and tight. About 20% of pregnant women face inconvenience due to itchy skin which starts in the stomach region and then spreads all over the body.

Itchiness

- Some areas of your skin may itch because they are dry and flaky; other areas may itch because of a prickly heat rash.

- The itch may be restricted to your abdomen region or it can again spread to other body parts. Patches of dry, red flaky rash may appear. The skin which has been stretched, is the most obvious reason for this – generally, this itching tends to subside after the baby is born.

Good to Know

Miscellaneous

- Healthy fats are good for baby's brain development. Try to add foods such as almonds, walnuts, avocados and salmon in moderation to your diet. That way you are kept feeling full longer as well.

- Women are more likely to crave for sweets during the second trimester than at any other point in pregnancy.

- The most active time for many babies is the 2nd half of the 7th month and the entire 8th month.

What is Cordocentesis Test?

- Cordocentesis is also called fetal blood or umbilical vein sampling.

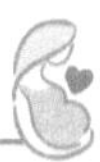

- This is an invasive procedure where fetal blood from the umbilical cord is taken and tested for suspected abnormalities.

- This diagnostic test can only be carried out between weeks 18-20 because before this time frame, baby's blood vessels are still fragile.

- Cordocentesis can be used to diagnose Down's Syndrome as a follow up to a scan.

- It helps in the detection of infections such as rubella, toxoplasmosis, herpes in the mother. A specific analysis is performed on the proteins found in the blood sample.

Wholesome Advice

- Studies indicate that babies will remember sounds that they have heard in the uterus and they have a preference for familiar sounds. Music you play now may help soothe the baby to sleep after birth.

- Make sure your diet contains plenty of B vitamins and good fats to support your baby's developing brain cells.

Your Actions Can Impact Your Baby's Growth

Managing migraines

- Migraines are fairly common in women of childbearing age. While some women get better after the first trimester, others continue to get more frequent and intense headaches. Now that you are pregnant migraine medicines are not advisable.

- Try sleeping it off in a quiet dark room and apply a cold compress to the forehead or neck.

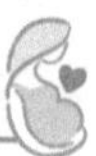

- Splash cold water on your face and back of the neck if a cold shower is not possible.

- Avoid offending foods such as MSG, chocolate, cheese, cured meats, etc. Keep your stomach full and blood sugar up, but avoid sugary foods in excess as this may cause blood sugar to rise rapidly and then crash.

- Stay active, get plenty of rest (catnaps to feel rested and relaxed), stick to regular sleep timings and avoid stress.

Herbal and all-natural supplements

- Many pregnant women resort to herbal and botanical products taking them to be safe since they are natural or organic. However, safely of such products is in question when it comes to pregnancy. Findings on herbal and botanical supplements are not conclusive enough to suggest that they are fine on a growing fetus and whether they are safe for consumption during pregnancy. You should check out each one and speak to your doctor before taking such supplements.

Common Concerns

What does 'small for dates' mean?

- This simply means baby is smaller than expected for the stage of pregnancy. Several reasons attribute to this. A lower amount of amniotic fluid will make the mother appear smaller although the baby is the right size. Maternal height, shape and abdominal muscles can also affect measurement.

- The fact that babies grow at different rates but are measured against averages has to be considered too. Some babies appear small for a while and then go through a growth spurt.

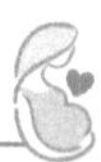

- 'Small for dates' can also indicate IUGR, a problem in which the placenta is not doing its job well. Ultrasound will usually be conducted to measure different parts of the baby's anatomy and a rescan 2 weeks later to determine baby's growth pattern. Adequate rest is important as it increases placental blood flow.

What is fundal height measurement?

- Fundal height measurement measures the upper edge of your pubic bone to the top of your uterus in centimeters. The measurement should equal the number of weeks of pregnancy, with a variation of 2 cm. Some women expecting their second or subsequent babies can measure slightly large for dates. If the measurement does not appear within the normal range, an ultrasound may be recommended.

Nutrition

- Iron is important during pregnancy; about 30 mg a day is required to meet the increased needs caused by the increase in blood volume.

- Your baby draws on your iron store to create its own storage for the first few months of life.

- Most prenatal vitamins contain sufficient iron to meet your needs. If you must take supplements, you can have it with a glass of orange juice or grapefruit juice to increase its absorption.

- Avoid drinking milk, coffee, tea or colas when taking iron supplements or when eating iron rich foods. They prevent the body from absorbing iron it needs.

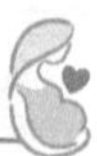

- If you feel tired, have problems concentrating, suffer from headaches, dizziness or indigestion or if you get sick easily, you may have an iron deficiency.

- An easy way to check is to examine the insides of your lower eyelid. If you are getting enough iron, it should be dark pink. Your nail beds should be pink too.

- Only 10-15% of the iron you consume is absorbed by the body. Your body stores it properly but you need to restock it daily to maintain the stores.

- Combining a vitamin C food and an iron rich food ensures better absorption by the body. A spinach salad with orange juice is a good example.

- Your prenatal vitamin contains about 60mg of iron. If you eat a well balanced diet and take your prenatal vitamin daily, you will not need to rely on supplements. Still, discuss with your doctor if you have any concerns.

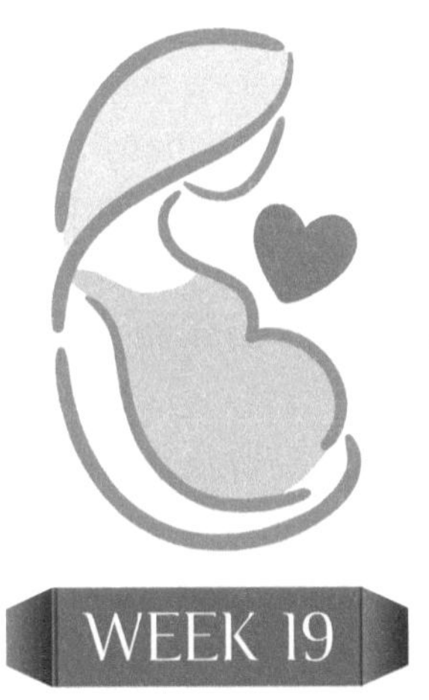

WEEK 19

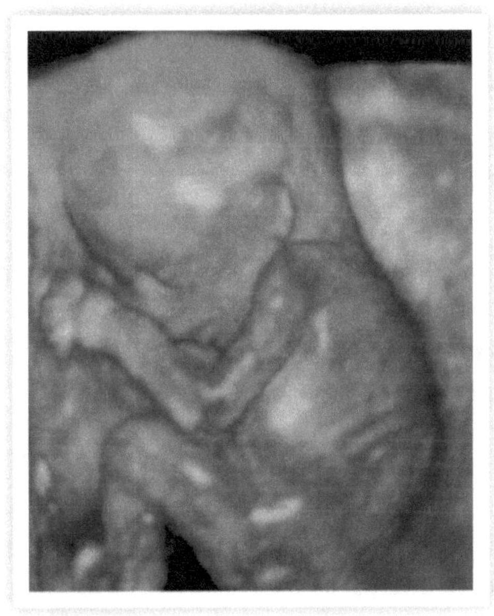

FOETUS AGE 17 WEEKS

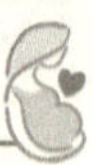

Changes in Baby

- From crown to rump, your baby measures at 5-6 inches and weighs about 7oz. Fetus is the size of an apple.

- This week, baby's skin becomes covered with vernix, the white, slippery, fatty coating that provides protection against chapping.

- Under the vernix is the fine down-like hair called lanugo which covers the skin.

- The kidneys are developed enough to make urine this week, which is secreted into the amniotic sac.

- Baby's hearing is well developed now - it may be able to hear your conversations!

- The brain is developing millions of motor neurons, nerves that help the brain muscles to communicate.

- Your baby may already have a preference for the left or right hand.

- In the brain, the nerve cells that serve the senses of touch, taste, smell, sight and hearing are forming complex connections - loud sounds or any feelings of stress may be communicated to the fetus. Baby responds by becoming more active.

Changes in You

- You may experience back pain as the weight of your expanding uterus causes your back to work harder at keeping you upright.

- Bulges start to show - bigger breasts and the bump above your pelvis.

- You still find yourself worrying that something could go

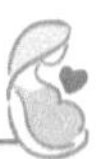

wrong, although the first trimester is over i.e. when your pregnancy is most vulnerable!

* In the next week or so, you will have an ultrasound to check your baby's organs.

Good to Know

* Back pain is mostly associated with the third trimester. Unfortunately, it often strikes in the second trimester even though you are not that big yet. Your pelvis is expanding and the ligaments supporting your abdomen are softening causing the joints between your pelvic joints to soften as well. That's why the backache!

Embryonic and fetal facts

* Each egg chooses the sperm it mates i.e. the egg opens its shell and welcomes the sperm it is attracted to.

* Unborn babies feel pain as powerfully as those outside the womb.

* The fetal heart beats for the very first time between days 22-25 after fertilization.

* Between weeks 28 and 32 your baby is capable of feeling and remembering.

* You need 75,000 calories to create a baby, of which sufficient amount is already stored as fat in your body to get you through the first trimester without the need to increase your calorie intake.

Chickenpox in pregnancy

* Chickenpox is a common childhood viral infection afflicting most of us, and unfortunately the most contagious of the lot. If you are pregnant, try to keep

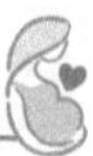

away from possible sources of infection because chickenpox in pregnancy can bring harm to your unborn child, especially if you are not immune to it. The comforting news is, once you have had chickenpox you cannot become infected with it again.

Wholesome Advice

* Low-fat, low-carb foods and most sugar substitutes have unhealthy chemicals. Though you wish to keep off the extra kilos, you need your carbohydrates and the full effects of sugar substitutes are not known. Therefore, plain old sugar in moderation is the best.

* If you find yourself getting irritable for no good reason, try a snack. Low blood sugar can make you tired and irritated.

Your Actions Can Impact Your Baby's Growth

The importance of water

* Your organs need water in order to function.

* Water is needed to make the plasma, an essential part of blood. Since blood volume has expanded, more plasma will be made, requiring more water.

* Water is needed to form the amniotic fluid.

* Waste needs to be flushed out by water.

* Water can help prevent bladder infections.

* Water helps urine stay diluted, hence reducing the chance for bladder infection.

* Drinking plenty of water wards off constipation.

* The more water you drink, the less likely you are to be bothered by a swollen body.

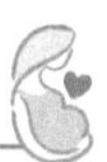

Omega-3 Fish Oil

- There are two types of fish oil supplements - those derived from fish liver and those made from fish body.

- Supplements from liver such as cod liver oil contain retinol, a form of vitamin A. It needs to be either totally avoided or consumed in careful dosage (should not exceed 3300 mcg).

- Fish oils derived from fish bodies are important for the formation of baby's eyes and brain. It is important to choose a version that is suited to pregnancy.

Common Concerns

Should I try harder at not giving in to my food cravings?

- It all depends on your cravings. If you crave for sugary foods and fatty foods, go ahead and indulge if the craving is rather strong. But bear in mind the nutrients your growing baby needs and try to work them into your sugar or salt fix. In other words eat in moderation.

Are there ways to control unhealthy food cravings?

- Eat breakfast everyday! This will help you cut back on mid-morning junking.

- Exercise regularly. A good walk for instance will help keep boredom and anxiety at bay.

- Get the emotional support you need right now; pregnancy makes you vulnerable to mood swings which can lead to snacking or comfort foods.

- Eat small portions and that includes your craved foods. Eat few spoonfuls of ice cream or pieces of chocolate instead of the entire tub or bar.

- Don't indulge everyday - see it as a treat once in a while.

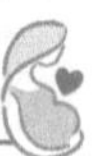

Intrauterine growth restriction

* Intrauterine growth restriction or IUGR is when your baby's estimated weight is below the 10th percentile for his gestational age.

The Risks...

* Premature labor

* Shortage of oxygen reaching baby at birth

* Neurological problems for baby after birth

Herbal use in pregnancy

* In the past, some of you may have used herbs and botanicals in the forms of teas, pills or powders to treat various ailments. Now that you are pregnant, it is advisable to not treat yourself with herbal remedies without asking your doctor first.

* You may think herbal remedy is safe and therefore fine to use, but it could be dangerous during pregnancy.

* For example, it you are constipated, you may decide to use senna, a herb, as a laxative. However, senna may stimulate uterine muscles causing you to miscarry.

* Some herbs may irritate your bowels and baby's bowels too. So play it safe - be extremely careful with any substances your doctor has not specifically recommended for you. Always check with your doctor before you decide on any step or action.

Nutrition

Pay attention to Calcium

* It is very important to get enough calcium every day. You need 1200mg daily - 50% more than your pre-pregnancy days.

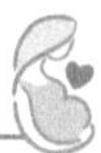

Sugar during pregnancy

- The best sugars are complex sugars (its complexity owing to the molecules being larger). Also referred to as complex carbs, the foods rich in this include pasta, potatoes, grains and seeds. Healthier sugars are the fructose sugars with fruits being the chief source. Lactose sugar is derived from dairy products. Both fructose and lactose provide you with quick energy and do not cause mood swings that simple sugars do. Simple sugars are the least nutritional; simple because the molecules are so small that they pass through into the bloodstream rather quickly. Blood sugar rises and triggers the release of insulin which brings down the blood sugar quickly. Sucrose, dextrose, glucose are some forms and most commercial foods containing them.

DHA (Docosahexaenoic Acid)

- DHA is considered the building block of the brain. DHA is one of the derivatives of Omega-3 Essential Fatty Acid (EFA). DHA has been recognized to enhance mental and visual development in babies and also plays a pivotal role in brain function. During pregnancy, from the final trimester onwards, DHA is taken up by the placenta and travels directly to the fetus's brain and retinal tissue.

- Omega-3 EFA is very essential for healthy development of brain, eyes and nervous tissue in the fetus and infant.

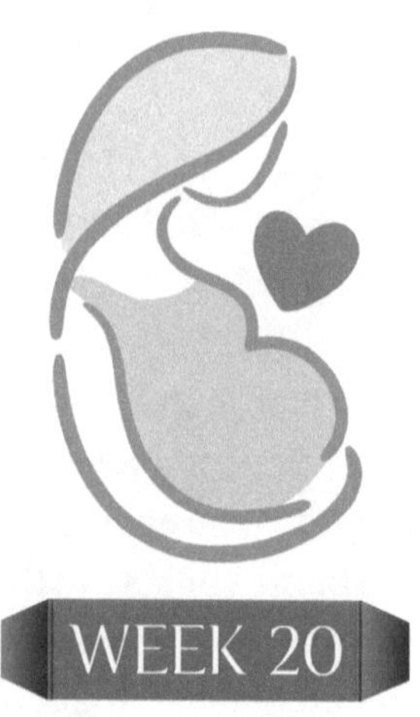

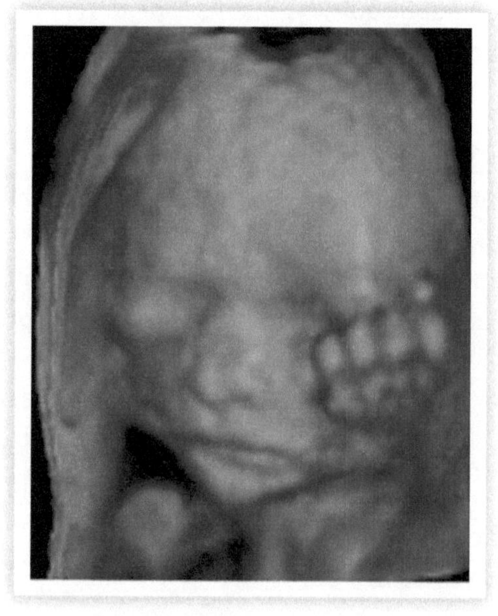

FOETUS AGE 18 WEEKS

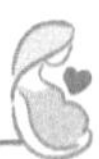

Changes in Baby

- From crown to rump, your baby measures at 6½ inches, weighs about 9oz or 255gm and is the size of a mango.

- Baby's permanent teeth are starting to form behind its baby teeth.

- Baby's legs are beginning to stretch out more instead of lying in a curled position.

- Baby's is starting to produce meconium, a dark colored by-product of digestion which will accumulate in baby's bowels.

- From this point onwards, baby seems to be able to differentiate between mornings, afternoons and nights by becoming more active at certain times more than others.

- Your baby has now all the neurons that it will need.

- Baby will be more active and flexible this trimester.

Changes in You

- You have made it to the halfway mark finally!

- You uterus is continuing to expand - by 20th week it will reach your navel.

- Sleeping problems are commonplace during pregnancy and get more obvious as the times goes by.

- Around now, you may feel a pulling and stabbing pain in your groin or a sharp cramp down your sides, more so after making a sudden move. This is round ligament pain, which although painful, is harmless.

- By the time you reach this point you probably would have gained about 10 pounds.

- Iron deficiency anemia develops most often after 20

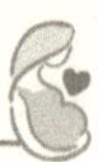

weeks of pregnancy. It can make you tired and more prone to illness.

- Adjust your diet to prevent heartburn or indigestion which may interfere with your sleep. Use pillows to support your bump.

- Your growth will now be monitored by measuring the height of your uterus with the tape measure - your uterus is now in line with your belly button. From now on, the growth at the top of your uterus will add at a rate of 1 cm a week.

Good to Know

Thongs

- Some studies show that thongs may increase the risk of bacterial vaginosis and UTI during pregnancy. You don't have to discontinue it's use if you have no discomfort or problems.

Fundus

- The growth rate of the uterus is more regular now. Your doctor will measure the size of your uterus from the pubic bone to the top of your uterus or fundus to gauge pregnancy progress. The distance is measured in cm and should be equal to the number of weeks you are, plus or minus 2 cm. If the measurements are not consistent for 2 weeks, the doctor will arrange for an ultrasound to rule out discrepancies.

Myelination

- This is the growth of myelin in the brain; it is a substance that acts like an electrical insulator of the systems that send messages between parts of the brain. The coating of

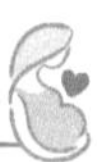

myelin keeps the wiring of the brain from crossing signals. A slow process, it begins now and continues through the first year of baby's life. The myelin composes of about 80% fat in babies diets and 20% protein - that is why pediatricians advise a high level of fats in babies diet until about age 2.

Wholesome Advice

- Dry hair will need extra conditioning during your pregnancy months because it becomes drier as hormonal changes occur. Conversely, oily hair may become greasier. Whatever the condition, try using milk shampoo preferably.

- As you get bigger, comfort becomes the key issue. Underwear can be worn above or below your waistline though over-the-belly offers comfort. Maternity versions come with spandex to provide support to your tummy below.

- You shouldn't just sleep on the left side because that is best for your baby. Relax and lie on whichever side that is comfortable.

Your Actions Can Impact Your Baby's Growth

Safe Traveling

- The two key issues to consider during travel are UTI and blood clots in the legs. UTI is more common during pregnancy, and more likely to increase if you sit for long periods without taking frequent breaks to flex your leg muscles. Reduce the stress of UTI by walking to the washroom a couple of times whether you are traveling by road or air.

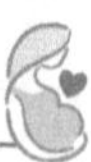

- It is proven that pregnant women are more prone to develop blood clots because pregnancy alters the coagulation factor in blood. The note of caution here is if the blood clot dislodges and makes its way to the lungs, it causes a deadly pulmonary embolus. The solution is simple, stretch your legs and exercise the muscles in your legs to maintain the flow.

- Always fasten your seatbelt if in a car journey - it is always safer for a pregnant mother to be belted. If involved in any road mishap, however small, it is best to get a thorough evaluation. Make it a point to take breaks and visit the washroom and stretch those legs.

- Fly only in a commercial pressurized cabin. Drink plenty of fluids and walk down the aisle a couple of times. Most airlines require a note from your doctor after week 32 of pregnancy. Once you are within a month of your due date, it is advisable to restrict your travel as this is the time you are most likely to go into labor. Various complications can occur now as well. Your prenatal visits are more frequent - once or twice a week, so it is best to stay on home grounds.

Brain Work

- Now is the time when your baby's brain is developing and a good time for you to ensure you are getting adequate fat. You need to make sure you are getting some amount of real non-hydrogenated fat in your diet.

- Omega-3 fatty acids found in oily fish such as salmon, tuna and sardines are good for your baby's brains. However, limit the intake to about 12 oz or 340 grams a week because of possible high mercury content.

- You can include fats in nuts, avocados and olive oil and the fats from dairy products. Try limiting your fat intake to one-third of your daily calories.

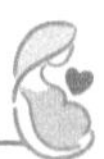

Common Concerns

Is it normal to have aches in the lower abdomen?

• It is normal to go through this - the aches are caused by the stretched muscles and ligaments that support your uterus. You are likely to experiences this mostly when you cough or get up from a seated position.

• What you need to do is rest - sit down, place your feet up and relax. Flexing your knees towards your abdomen provides you the relief as well.

• Alternatively, you can lie down on either side with a pillow tucked under your belly and another between your legs.

• If the pain is severe with cramps, bleeding, fever or a feeling of faintness, please alert your doctor.

Should I be eating lots of dairy products now that I am in my 2nd trimester?

• It all depends on how much you normally intake. Dairy products are a excellent source of calcium, protein, vitamin D and phosphorus - all essential for baby's growth and development in areas like bones and teeth, heart and nerves and blood clotting as well.

• Aim to eat 3-4 servings of calcium rich foods a day during your pregnancy, enough to give you an 1000 mg. Opt for low or non-fat dairy products - you will benefit from all the necessary nutrients without the excess fats.

I feel more comfortable sharing my pregnancy concerns with my girlfriend than my partner - is this normal?

• Many women don't feel totally understood by their partners during their pregnancies. They feel more comfortable talking to their female counterpart

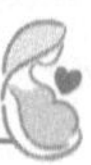

i.e. friend, sister or mother. A man tends to have a different perspective and this is largely to do with him having no comprehension on the minute details and feelings of being pregnant. So while it is perfectly normal to share your pregnancy with your girlfriend, there are other ways your partner can participate and be a part of your pregnancy.

Nutrition

* Magnesium is an important mineral during pregnancy, Magnesium during pregnancy helps prevent many health concerns from cropping up such as heart disease, diabetes and high blood pressure. However, magnesium in the pregnant months isn't sufficiently emphasized and so this mineral doesn't get its due attention.

* Many women use artificial sweeteners to help cut calories. Aspartame is the most commonly available in the market. Saccharin, not so popular today, is also added to many foods and beverages. Aspartame is a combination of phenylalanine and aspartic acid, two amino acids. It is advisable that you substitute foods that do not contain these sweeteners.

* If you suffer from phenylketonuria, you must follow a low-phenylalanine diet or your baby will suffer adverse effects. In all other situations, limit your use of artificial sweeteners if you cannot help it. If you can avoid them, do not resort to artificial sweeteners. It is probably best to totally eliminate any substances you can do without from the food you eat and beverages you drink.

* Sucralose is another type of sweetener, and it is derived from sugar. Sucralose passes through the body without

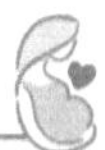

being metabolized - your body does not recognize it as either sugar or carbohydrates which is what makes sucralose, low calorie. Surcralose is used in salad dressings, baked goods, desserts, dairy products, beverages, jams, jellies, coffee and tea syrups. Sucralose is safe for pregnant and nursing women to use.

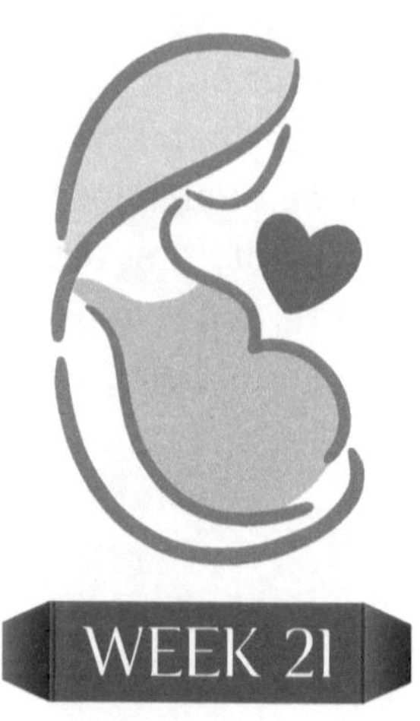

WEEK 21

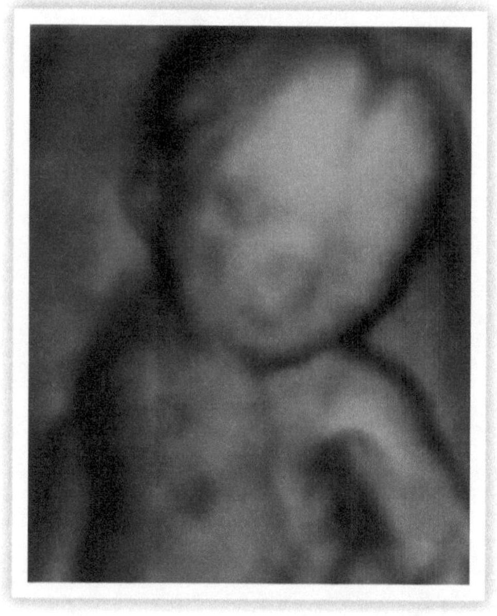

FOETUS AGE 19 WEEKS

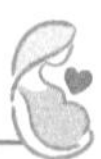

Changes in Baby

* From crown to rump, your baby measures at 7 inches and weighs about 10½ oz. Fetus is now the length of a spoon.

* Growth rate has slowed down - weight gain for baby is more sure and steady now.

* All the body systems will mature at a gradual pace.

* Baby swallows amniotic fluid to prepare the digestive system for functioning after birth. Any unabsorbed material in the fluid becomes the meconium in baby's intestinal tract.

* Baby regularly drinks amniotic fluid for hydration and nutrition, urinates in the fluid and breathes in and out. The fluid pool is replenished with fresh stock every 3 hours.

* Baby's eyebrows and eyelids are fully formed; although the eyelids are sealed, the eyes are active.

* Taste buds are beginning to form on baby's tongue.

* Bone marrow is starting to make blood cells.

Changes in You

* Time has come to say goodbye to your waistline.

* Blood vessels in your breasts are continuing to be more visible.

* At 21 weeks, the hormones progesterone and oestrogen will be at par and by 24th week the oestrogen level will be slightly higher.

* Your blood pressure will continue to stay lower than normal this week.

* If you are getting enough iron, production of red blood

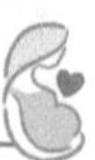

cells should be catching up to production of plasma. If not, the risk of developing iron deficiency anemia will rise.

- Nasal congestion, nose bleeds and bleeding gums are commonplace. These are due to continued increased blood flow to the nasal passages and gums.

- You may gain 1½ pounds this week and only ½ pound the next, but this is no cause for concern. Weight gain should be steady without drastic changes.

Good to Know

In General

- Your blood pressure reaches its lowest levels during the second trimester. If you get lightheaded, stand still and let it pass. If it doesn't pass, sit down and put your head between your knees.

- Braxton Hicks contractions (false labor) start around now. Each contraction can last for a few minutes to several minutes.

Smooth Muscles

- Your body has three types of muscles: skeletal, cardiac and smooth. Muscle changes impact your pregnancy, causing everything from constipation to vision changes.

- Pregnancy has the most effect on smooth muscles which are found in your uterus, stomach bowels, in the iris of your eyes and in hair follicles. This kind of muscle is not under your voluntary control.

- Some smooth muscles relax their functions during pregnancy, like the ones in your bowels. The smooth muscles in your arteries also relax causing your vessels

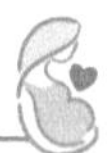

to widen and in turn lower your blood pressure and more blood then flows into the placenta.

• Smooth muscles also regulate contractions during labor; first the falsies in the form of Braxton Hicks contractions and eventually the real ones to help in the birth of your baby.

Wholesome Advice

• If this is your first pregnancy and you are not sure of the difference between the real contraction and Braxton Hicks, do not ignore contractions that intensify and increase in frequency. This can be a sign of premature labor.

• Start educating and preparing yourself early, on either medication or relaxation techniques to help you deal with labor.

• If local water is an issue when you are traveling, avoid ice cubes in restaurants. Avoid tap water. Choose canned or bottled drinks; make sure the bottles you buy are sealed. You can also treat water with water purifying tablets or by boiling and filtering it.

Your Actions Can Impact Your Baby's Growth

Fiber

• Fiber is not digested by your body - it passes through and helps to alleviate constipation. Both soluble (oat bran, beans, peas and psyllium husk) and insoluble fibers (whole wheat products) are required. Soluble fibers absorb liquid and form a gel while insoluble fibers dont. Most fruits and vegetables contain both.

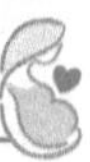

Psyllium

- This is a safe fiber supplement - it is not a laxative. You can buy psyllium without additives, dies and sugar versions from health food stores. Start slowly once a day for a few days. Work your way up to twice a day if you see no improvement.

Falls

- Since you are more prone to falls, now that there are changes in your center of gravity, learning to reduce the likelihood of falling with certain precautions is helpful during your normal daily life:
  - Avoid high heels
  - Walk on pathways whenever you can
  - Avoid uneven surfaces or stony paths
  - Wear appropriate footwear whenever you work out

- If you do fall, do not panic. Check yourself out thoroughly before standing back up. Mostly, remember that your baby is well cushioned by the amniotic bag. However, in the event of any abdominal pain, bleeding, contractions or changes in baby's movements, inform your doctor immediately.

Common Concerns

Should contact lenses be a concern during pregnancy?

- Water retention can change the shape of your eyeball and therefore the fit of the lenses. It is worth getting your eyesight and fit of your lenses checked out. If your eyesight is changing, you might want to considered disposable lenses so that the prescription can be changed more quickly and economically throughout

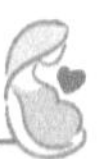

your pregnancy. If you suffer from dry eyes, you may want to limit the time you wear your lenses and use your glasses in between. If you have blurred vision and flashing lights, check this out with your doctor before seeing your optician as the cause maybe something more serious such as gestational diabetes.

Will flying harm my baby?

* There is no evidence suggesting this to be a fact. Heavy exposure to atmospheric radiation during flying has been linked to an increased risk of miscarriage and Down's Syndrome and for this reason it is not advisable to fly during the first trimester. However, the risk to females who only fly occasionally is negligible.

Are airport screening machines safe?

* They use low level metal detectors, so they are safe. The same holds true for wands that are passed over passengers. Many people think these machines take x-rays - they don't. Airport x-ray machines are used only on luggage.

Nutrition

* Some women experience cravings during pregnancy. Food cravings have been long considered a non-specific sign of pregnancy.

* Cravings can be good and bad. If the food you crave for is nutritious and healthful, eat in moderation. If you crave for foods high in fat and sugar or loaded with empty calories, watch out! Indulge a little bit, but don't let yourself go.

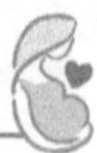

- Try substituting with something more nourishing such as a fruit or low-calorie flavored yoghurt instead of giving in to your craving.

- Hormonal and emotional changes are responsible for cravings.

- On the reverse side of the coin is food aversion. Some foods that you used to enjoy before becoming pregnant now make you sick in the stomach. This is common.

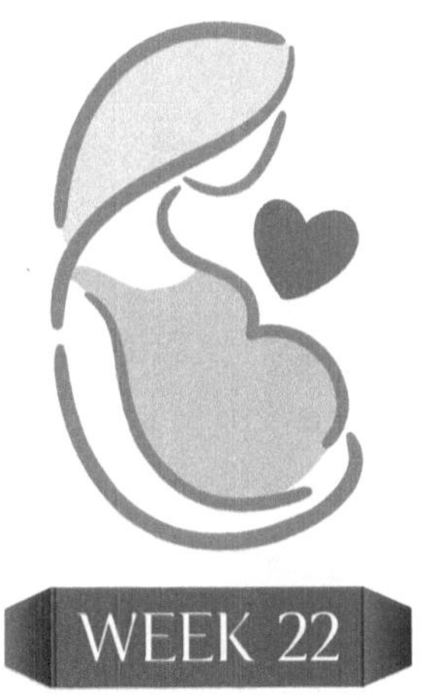

WEEK 22

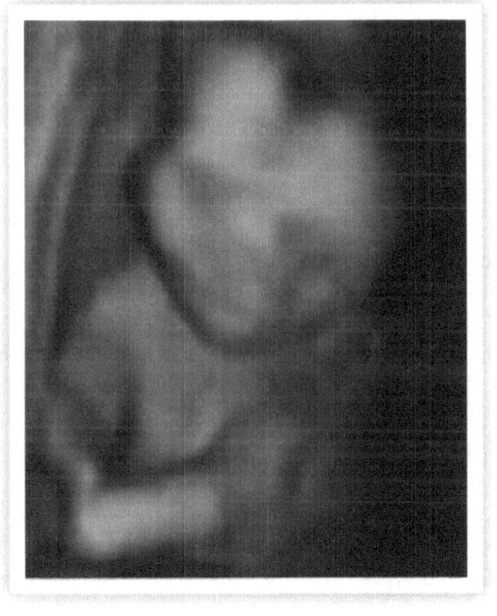

FOETUS AGE 20 WEEKS

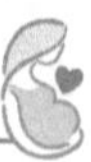

Changes in Baby

- From crown to rump, your baby measures at 7½ inches and weighs about 13-16 oz. Fetus is now the size of a grapefruit.

- Baby has now entered its fifth month of existence.

- Fingernails are almost fully grown.

- Baby's organ functions are more specialized.

- Baby now looks like a miniature newborn.

- If you could have a sneak preview, you might see your baby experimenting with its newfound sense of touch - feeling its face or other parts of its body.

- With a boy baby, the testes are beginning to descend from his abdomen this week.

- With a girl baby, the uterus and ovaries are now in place and her vagina is developed.

Changes in You

- Though your uterus is growing, you are still comfortable with bending over, sitting and driving at this stage.

- You may have increased vaginal discharge (thin, white discharge with no odour) which may sometimes develop into yeast infections.

- To accommodate your increasing lung capacity, your rib cage is growing larger as well and by the time baby is born your rib cage will have expanded by 2-3 inches. It will return to its pre-pregnancy size after baby is born.

- Your lower spine continues to curve backward to help prevent you from falling forward because of the weight of the growing baby.

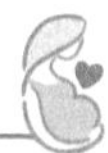

- This period on, fears about the process of giving birth will occupy your thoughts.

Good to Know

Miscellaneous

- At full term, your baby can swallow as much as 500 ml of amniotic fluid in a 24 hour period.

- Striae gravidarum are the stretch marks that all pregnant women dread. About 50% of all pregnant women get them. The only thing that can absolutely prevent them are genetics!

- Though baby's eyes are developed, it's iris still has no colour.

Wholesome Advice

- A full body pillow is one of the great inventions for pregnancy. Many maternity stores carry them, or your other option is to shop online.

- Treat yourself to a maternity massage. It's good for the body and mind. Avoid lying on your back. A therapist qualified in pregnancy massage is important – check beforehand.

- Products like cocoa butter, mango butter and olive oil won't prevent stretch marks, but they smell nice and they provide relief against the itches. Good old lotion will help the itching just as well. Use a lot of it.

- The swelling (edema) is most noticeable during the second half of the pregnancy.

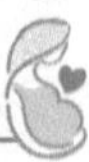

Things you can do...

- Drink lots of water to help flush excess fluids, toxins from your system; drinking more will reduce retention.

- Stay active - move about and do some light exercises like walking to keep your blood pumping.

- Don't add salt to your food and check the salt content of everything you eat.

- Sit down with your legs raised up, or better still, lie down on your left side when you feel like resting.

- Try wearing support tights that are waste high; this keeps your circulation in check.

- Avoid socks or stockings that constrict at the ankle or calves.

Your Actions Can Impact Your Baby's Growth

Overheated

- During pregnancy your metabolism or the rate at which your body expends energy speeds up. You are also perspiring more, due to needing to lose all the heat your baby is making. This can make you feel rather warm even in cooler temperatures. It is very important to stay cool while you are pregnant.

- Drink plenty of water and fluids. In fact, carry a water bottle with you.

- Dress lightly in breathable fabrics like cotton.

- Stay out of the sun as much as possible.

- Stay in an air-conditioned environment if the heat gets too much.

- Go for a swim or take cool baths or showers.

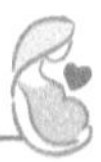

- Avoid exercising in the warmest part of the day. Take a walk when the sun is down i.e. early morning or evening, or go to the fitness centre for a workout.

Yeast Infections

- Increased estrogen levels during pregnancy cause changes in the vaginal environment which throws off the natural balance and makes room for some organisms to multiply faster than others. Candida may be present without symptoms and may cause an infection. Signs of vaginal infection include thick, white and curd-like discharge; itching, redness around the vaginal area and burning sensation when urinating. Though unpleasant for you, it will not harm your baby and it is treatable during pregnancy. Help prevent yeast infections with these measures:

  - Eat yoghurt that contains live Lactobacillus Acidophilus cultures. It helps maintain the right mix of bacteria in your system.

  - Wear underwear with cotton crotches and loose fitting pants that do not cut into your crotch area.

  - Avoid sugar laden foods as these encourage bacterial growth.

  - Avoid long hot baths which create the perfect environment for yeast to flourish. Opt for showers instead.

  - Avoid wearing wet bathing suits and exercise gear for long periods of time; wash them after each use.

  - Do not self treat with remedies available over the counter. Consult your doctor.

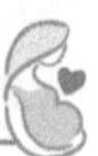

Common Concerns

Is a small breast lump of concern in the 5th month of pregnancy?

- Since the breast are collections of glands that make milk, it is not unusual for a milk duct to get engorged - this happens frequently. It is possible that a breast lesion becomes more prominent and obvious during pregnancy. Since it is difficult to draw a line between what is suspicious and unsuspicious, the following will help you decide on what is unsuspicious:

  - Freely movable (cancerous cells tend to stick in the surrounding tissue).

  - Painful, which usually means inflammation, not tumor. It is possible to get mastitis before actual breastfeeding begins.

  - Size - cysts related to milk production change size with hormonal fluctuations. Bad cycts will stay the same or grow bigger.

  - Very round (malignant growths are irregularly shaped).

  - Small size (less than 1cm).

  - Breast lumps are fairly common during pregnancy. Mammogram, if necessary is safe, especially if an abdominal shield is used and any procedure following that is best left at your obstetrician's discretion.

There is some fluid coming from my breasts staining my clothes. I am only half-way through my pregnancy - is this breast milk?

- This isn't breast milk. During the second trimester a thin, yellow fluid called colostrum forms, which is a precursor

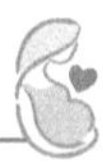

to breast milk. Sometimes it will leak from the breasts and this is normal. It is usually best to leave your breast alone; don't try to squeeze the fluid out. Wear breast pads if necessary.

Nutrition

- Fluids, especially water is very important during pregnancy - its importance cannot be emphasized enough.

- We tend to forget or ignore our thirst, but the fact remains that fluids help your body process nutrients, develop new cells, keep up blood volume and regulate body temperature.

- Studies indicate that for every 15 calories your body burns, you need 1 tablespoon of water; for 2000 calories you will need about 2 quarts of water.

- Since your caloric needs increase during this time, so will your need for water.

- 6-8 glasses per day is good and this excludes beverages. Milk, vegetable juice, fruit juice and herbal teas are choices you can take besides water. Do not count tea, coffee or cola as fluids - in fact, avoid them.

- The sodium and caffeine in beverages function as diuretics.

- Common problems like headaches, constipation, bladder infections and uterine cramping become less of a problem if you are good in your fluid intake.

- Your urine is a good barometer to check on your intake. If it is light yellow to clear, you are doing fine; dark yellow on the other hand suggests that you have to up your intake.

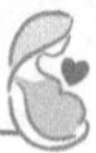

- Don't wait till you get thirsty to drink something; by that time you would have already lost 1% of your body's fluids. A good tip is to sip on fluids - water and juices - throughout the day and not only when you are thirsty.

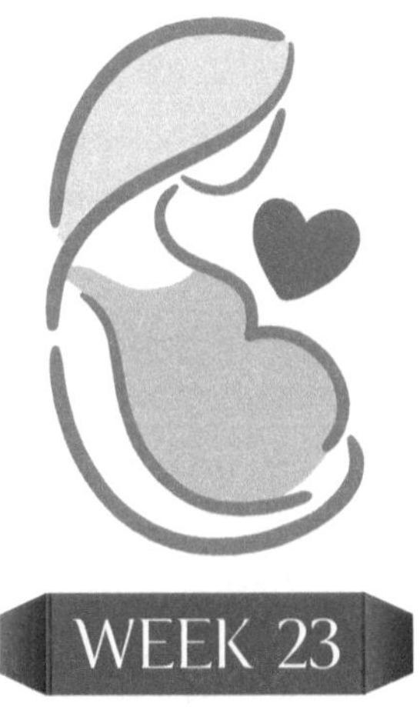

WEEK 23

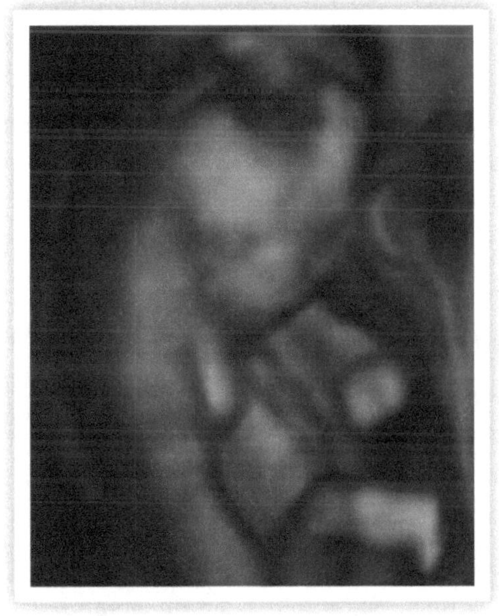

FOETUS AGE 21 WEEKS

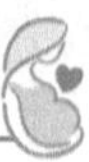

Changes in Baby

- From crown to rump, your baby measures at 8 inches and weighs about 1 pound. Fetus is now the size of a bag of coffee beans.

- First layers of fat are deposited, causing baby's skin to fill out; muscles are still growing.

- Your baby's lungs are developing rapidly this week - they are starting to produce the substance that lines the sac in the lungs (surfactant).

- Your baby is still receiving oxygen from the placenta - there is no air in the lungs until after birth.

- Although your baby resembles a baby, it is still frail and fragile with little body fat and wrinkled loose-hanging skin.

- The blood vessels in the brain are delicate and immature at 23 weeks.

Changes in You

Why dizzy spells during pregnancy?

- Occasionally, you may feel your head spinning. This is because your cardiovascular and nervous systems are not able to match up with the changes taking place in your body as you may have low BP.

- You feel faint when your brain is not able to get enough blood supply. Skipping a single meal will cause your blood sugar levels to drop and this will cause you to feel weak and lightheaded. Next thing you know, you have hit the ground. Fainting enables blood to reach your brain with greater immediacy. It is not the ideal solution, but

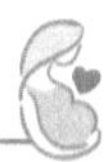

definitely effective. That is not to say that you should wait to fall when you feel dizzy.

* As your baby gains weight, so do you.

* With expansion, the tendency to itch grows more serious. Invest in any cream that smells good and absorbs well.

* Your doctor should be monitoring your expanding uterus and weight.

* As your size expands, you may want to keep a close watch on sodium which can make you sweat and bloat.

* Around this week, your uterus may begin practicing for labor and delivery; these warm up contractions called Braxton Hicks contractions are also called false labor.

* The ligaments supporting your abdomen are continuing to stretch and the joints between the pelvic bones are softening and loosening in preparation for childbirth.

Good to Know

In General

* Your baby's brain has begun to grow very quickly now, especially in the germinal matrix, a structure in the centre of the brain that manufactures brain cells. This structure disappears before birth. Your baby's brain continues to expand until the age of 5.

* One pound of what you are carrying now, is your baby.

* Fetal heart rate slows down when the mother is speaking, which suggests that fetus is calmed by your voice.

* Kegels exercise your pelvic floor muscles and keep them strong. Strong pelvic muscles will help you push your baby out and prevent major urine leakage after you have

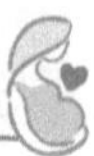

your baby. But, there is only so much Keggels can do. Despite 100 Kegels a day, every day, some women still pee a little when they sneeze or laugh.

Hepatitis B in pregnancy

• Hepatitis B, a viral infection that affects the liver is especially a concern during pregnancy, because it can be passed to the newborn at delivery. Hepatitis B can also be transmitted to the fetus if the pregnant lady is affected. Hepatitis B in pregnancy is linked to pre-term delivery to some extent.

Wholesome Advice

• If you are on your feet a lot, consider wearing a support hose or special stockings to help relieve the pressure on your legs.

• Typing on the keyboard can aggravate Carpal Tunnel Syndrome. Consider wearing a supportive wristband and investing in an ergonomic keyboard, if you haven't got one already.

• It is important that you stand up and sit with good alignment. Your lower back should be well supported and it should be more straight than curved. If you lift weights, or do aerobics, watch yourself in the mirror constantly to eye your stance.

Your Actions Can Impact Your Baby's Growth

Unpleasant truths about weight

• Gaining weight in pregnancy can lead to a progressive weight problem for a lot of women.

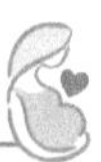

- After the baby is born, you will have a lot of issues to deal with and exercise and diet will probably not rank high in your list of priorities.

- Your metabolism slows down with age; you will not be able to shed the pounds as easily as you did earlier.

- Every pregnancy increases a woman's risk for obesity by 7% and her partner's by 4%.

- Weight loss by pregnancy may not work for you - while breastfeeding can burn 500 calories per day, it also makes you really hungry.

- Exercise alone is not enough; you will have to work real hard at cutting calories.

Overweight and Pregnant

- An obese mother can make it 3½ times more likely for her baby to be born with spina bifida and 3 times more likely for the baby to be born with a defect known as omphalocele (the defect causes the intestines to protrude through the navel). Researchers suspect the link between obesity and these birth defects is a diet high in empty calories and low in vitamins.

- Women who gain more than 40 pregnancy pounds also increase the risk of post-menopausal breast cancer by 63%.

- If your BMI is 30 or higher, consider getting medical help.

Women who exercise on the average:

- Gain less excess weight and therefore are less likely to suffer from complications.

- Have shorter labors.

- Have fitter babies.

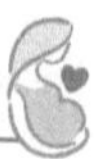

- Retain less fluid.
- Sleep better and feel more energized.
- Have bodies that regulate their temperature and use oxygen more efficiently.
- Have lower risk of injuries from accidents. Woman who do not exercise suffer from strains and sprains.
- Are less likely to suffer from depression.
- Physically recover faster after childbirth.
- Are less likely to suffer from falls.

Common Concerns

I am experiencing conflict in emotions about my pregnancy. Is this normal?

- It is very normal to feel this way. Such feelings arise from your adjustment to your pregnancy. You are heading towards a path of incredible changes that will involve many aspects of your life. Your feelings of conflict come from your attempt to deal with all the questions and concerns you have. This can happen if you are having your first baby or are expanding your family further.

Is it true that it is not unusual to experience pain in the uterus during pregnancy?

- As your uterus expands, you may start to feel slight cramping or even pain in your lower abdominal region on the sides. Your uterus tightens and contracts throughout your pregnancy. Some women don't go through this, which is also normal. However if the contractions are accompanied by bleeding from the vagina, alert your doctor immediately.

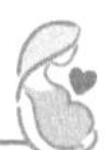

Nutrition

- You may have to watch your salt intake during pregnancy. Excess sodium causes water retention, leading to bloating and swelling.

- Avoid foods with high salt such as salted nuts, chips, pickles, canned foods and processed foods.

- Food labels will indicate the salt content per serving. However, some foods have no indications; like fast foods. You have to be careful with fast foods.

- Create the habit of reading labels before buying it off the shelf. Go easy on fast foods such as burgers and fries.

- Some foods with high salt content to give you an idea of what you are digging into:

Food serving	Portion	Sodium content (mg)
Salt	1 teaspoon	1938
Hamburger	1 regular	963
Cola	8 oz	16
Oatmeal	Cup	523
Potato chips	20 regular	400
Cottage cheese	1 cup	580
American cheese	1 slice	322

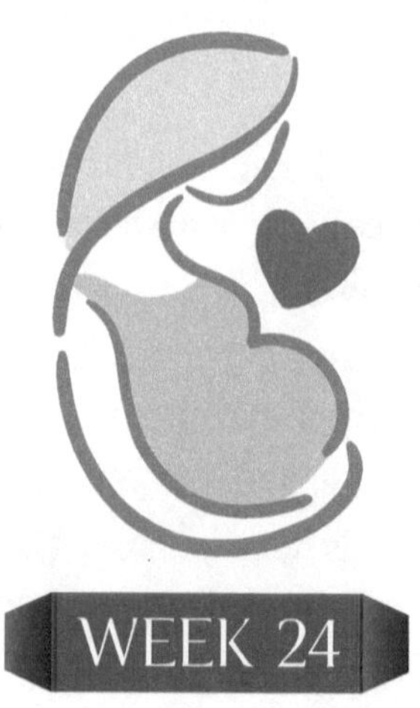

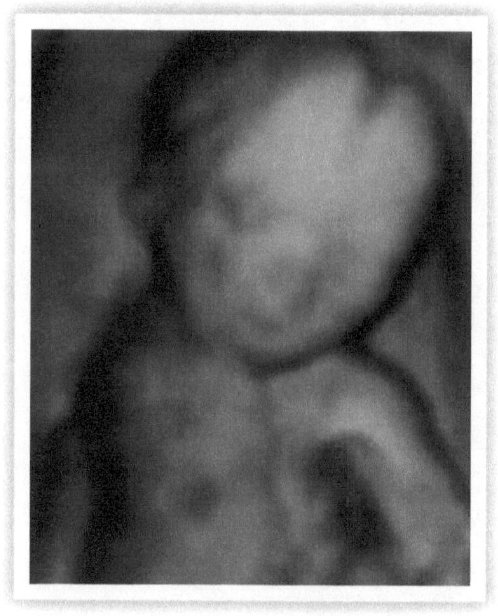

FOETUS AGE 22 WEEKS

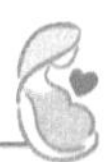

Changes in Baby

- From crown to rump, your baby measures at 8½ inches and weighs about 1 lb 6 oz. Fetus is now the size of a banana.

- All the main organs are working, except for the lungs, which baby will not use until after birth.

- Baby is becoming much more aware of its surroundings, sounds and movements outside the uterus.

- Your baby's unique hand and foot prints are forming.

- Baby's heart rate has dropped to about 140-150 beats a minute.

- The meconium of baby's first stool is starting to form in the bowel.

- Within the lungs, small air sacs or alveoli are forming.

- Sweat glands are forming in baby's skin.

- Baby is now able to cough and hiccup.

- Baby's skin is no more translucent, but reddish in color.

Changes in You

- Around this time, you may have a growth spurt, so your bump becomes more visible.

- The fundus is now above your belly button.

- When the baby moves, you may be able to make out a little foot or leg through the abdominal wall.

- Your body is retaining water, adding weight on your thighs and upper body.

- You may feel warmer these days.

- You may be suffering from heartburn, muscle aches, sore feet, fatigue and dizziness.

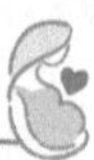

- Consult your doctor if dizzy spells are frequent as this may be a sign of anemia.

Glucose Screening Test during Pregnancy

- Gestational diabetes can develop even if you have no history of sugar-related problems in the family. It is good to find out earlier if you have this condition since your doctor will be able to guide you on a low-carb diet and exercise program. It is normally carried out between weeks 24-28 and performed earlier if there is a family history of diabetes or your routine urine test shows higher than normal glucose levels.

Good to Know

In General

- Apart from linea nigra and darkened areolas, pregnancy can make skin protrusions grow i.e. skin tags. Moles may grow in size or change. If a mole changes size, shape or color you need to have it checked just to be on the safe side.

Protein

- Urine sample at each prenatal visit will test for ketones, protein and glucose. Excessive protein or albumin in the urine can be a sign of preeclampsia. It is also a possible indication of UTI or renal (kidney) impairment. The presence of white blood cells also points to infection. Pregnant women typically excrete 260 mg of protein or less in a 24 hour period.

Ketone

- Ketones may appear in pregnancy if you are suffering

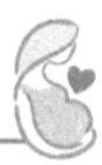

from severe nausea and vomiting. These substances are produced when the body is not getting sufficient fuel from food to metabolize fat for energy. This process results in ketones spilling into the urine.

Wholesome Advice

- If your neighborhood is being sprayed with bugs spray, stay inside with your windows shut. No one knows whether the sprays are safe for pregnant women or not. Since it can kill those bugs, it makes sense to be cautious.

- Antibiotics only work on bacterial infections and are useless against any viral infections. Don't take them unless you and your doctor are sure that a bacterial infection is the cause of your ailment.

- Finger and toe nails grow faster in pregnancy. This is a good time to go for a manicure or pedicure. If you have varicose veins, skip the calf massage routine.

Your Actions Can Impact Your Baby's Growth

Neck Spasm

- Weight gain during pregnancy can impact your posture. Pregnancy is also a stressful time and a lot of people react to stress by hunching their neck and shoulder muscles. Spasms can result if you are at your computer all day or don't move around enough on your job. You need to remind yourself to turn your head and roll your neck around to help avoid tension headaches and muscle pains. Neck pain is also caused by poor sleeping positions or by inactivity that comes with bed rest.

- Check your posture to see if you are sitting up straight from time to time; sit in a chair that lends support to your spine.

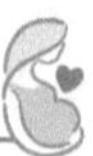

- Sit completely back in the chair and place a pillow for proper support if necessary.

- Support your feet on a footstool.

- Gentle heat pads and kneading on the affected areas and mild stretching helps.

- Check with your doctor for the most suitable pain reliever.

Carpal Tunnel Syndrome

- Around the 5th and 6th months of pregnancy, you may find pain, numbness, tingling and burning sensations in your wrists, fingers and even in your arms. This is most likely due to Carpal Tunnel Syndrome, a condition that often occurs in both hands of pregnant women. Excess fluid which your body is now retaining, presses against the median nerves in your arm and wrist. The carpal tunnel ligament is a tough membrane that holds the wrist bones together. Any swelling in the area can compress the median nerve. Temporary in nature, these pains go away after the baby is born.

- In the meanwhile, it helps if you wear a wrist splint at nights and during activities that make the symptoms worse such as typing, holding a book or when driving. Elevating your arms and hands help drain the fluid trapped in your tissues.

- Rub and shake your hands periodically.

- Soaking your wrists in warm water or resting them on a heating pad at night may help.

- Take frequent breaks if you are working on a keyboard for prolonged hours.

- Apply cold or hot compresses to the affected area.

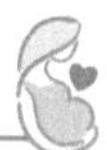

- Make sure your diet and prenatal vitamin has an adequate supply of vitamin B6 as studies show a link between this condition and a lack of this vitamin.

- In very severe cases, a minor surgery may be needed to rectify the problem.

Common Concerns

How do I know my baby is moving around enough?

- You will soon get to know your baby's pattern. Some babies are more passive - no one really knows if babies do vary in the amount they move. Movements are more obvious when you are resting. The most important factor is that you feel some movements from now onwards, if not earlier.

Why my bump is smaller than my friend's when our babies are due at the same time?

- Your baby is roughly the same size as your friend's baby at this point. Bump size depends on the amniotic fluid level, the amount of space inside your abdomen which is governed by your physical structure and overall size. Generally, bumps tend to be bigger in petite women than in women of bigger frames. If this is not your first baby, your bump will get bigger quicker because the uterus and abdomen have stretched in the past.

What are the signs of Preeclampsia?

- Preeclampsia is a complicated, dangerous pregnancy-related version of high blood pressure or hypertension. It can cause problems to both the mother and baby. The cause is not totally understood, but it tends to be genetic

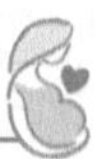

and there seems to be a link to the way the placenta grows, though this is not conclusive; strangely the symptom goes away once the placenta is delivered.

Nutrition

- If you are going to eat out, for now stick to foods or eateries that are familiar; chicken, salads, fish, fruits and vegetables are good choices. Avoid spicy fare.

- Eating out may also cause water retention problem in some of you. Besides spicy foods, avoid foods laden with salt, calories and foods such as fried foods, junk foods and rich desserts.

- Besides the calories, such foods won't settle too well on you. It is also very challenging to eat right when you eat out every day; working women are only too familiar with this problem.

- Look for healthy low-cal foods. For example request for steamed food instead of fried. Top-up your meals with fruit or vegetable or fruit juice.

Nuts and seeds during pregnancy

- Nuts and seeds during pregnancy are a good source of essential fatty acids, fiber, protein and minerals; including calcium. Some nuts are also a good source of folate. Nuts also contain useful plant chemicals. During pregnancy, nuts and seeds become a healthier alternative form of snacking.

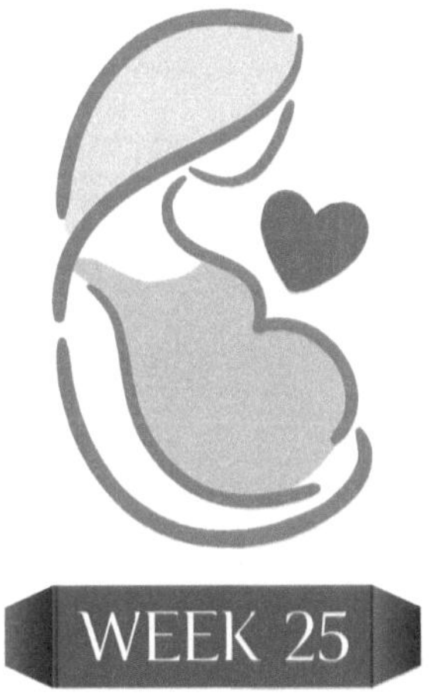

WEEK 25

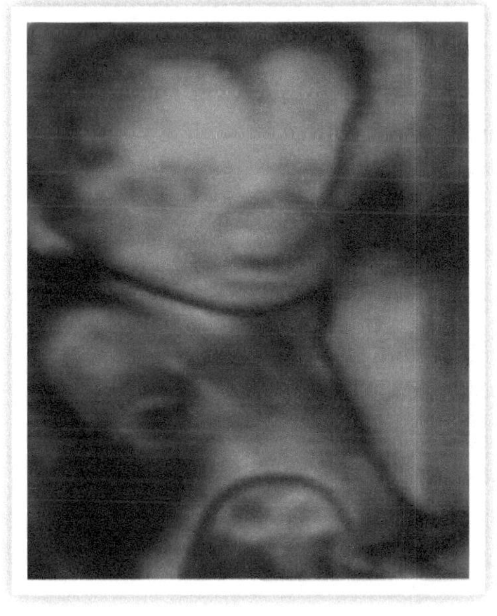

FOETUS AGE 23 WEEKS

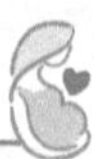

Changes in Baby

* From crown to rump, your baby measures at 9 inches and weighs about 1¼ pounds.

* Your baby can touch and hold its feet.

* Baby's nostrils which have been plugged, open up now.

* Baby is now beginning to explore its environment and structures inside the uterus

Changes in You

* You are now in your third trimester - with this comes fatigue, dizziness and frequent trips to the washroom.

* Your uterus is now the size of a soccer ball with your ribs, diaphragm and stomach; all compressed. This compression causes you to feel full after eating just a little food.

* With weight gain, chances for developing hemorrhoids rises.

* You may have cramps in your calves, back and tailbone as your ligaments soften.

* Your lung capacity is continuing to increase this month - this change allows your blood to carry oxygen in and carbon dioxide out at an increase rate. Breathing is slightly faster and experiencing some shortness of breath can be expected.

Good to Know

Miscellaneous

* Choose the right size of bra.

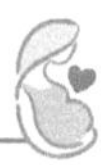

- During sex, be sure to move your legs around a lot or you might end up with a leg cramp.

- Just like stretch marks, varicose veins are genetic.

- High inside the gums, your baby's permanent teeth are forming in buds. These adult teeth won't descend until the baby teeth fall out at about age 6.

- Purplish or red veins on legs or abdomen which are painless, thin and spider-looking are spider veins; they usually disappear after birth. Varicose veins, on the other hand bulge and appear as thick and blue beneath the skin, mostly on the legs. The biggest difference is varicose can be quite painful during pregnancy.

- You may continue to have an increased vaginal discharge.

Your Breasts

- A pregnant woman's breasts contain many complex components: a network of nerves that respond to baby's suckling; fatty tissue that protects breasts from injury; glandular tissue; milk ducts that convert proteins and fats from blood into milk and ducts that deliver the milk to the nipples.

Wholesome Advice

- There isn't much you can do to prevent varicose veins other than avoid prolonged standing or lifting, wearing supportive stockings, putting your legs up whenever you can and going for short walks to aid in circulation.

- Now is a good time to be walking, swimming and practicing yoga, but avoid weightlifting or any exercises that might injure your softened ligaments.

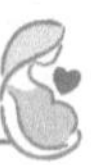

Your Actions Can Impact Your Baby's Growth

Sun Protection Lotions

- Sunscreen is safe to use during pregnancy. Pick one that is PABA (para-aminobenzoic acid) - free since PABA is known to cause skin irritation in some people.

- Sunless tanners are also considered safe but not a very good idea right now. Since skin pigment changes are happening now and increased perspiration and oil production are also occurring at the same time, what you will end up with is a blotchy skin.

Third Trimester Fatigue

- Fatigue and dizziness return in this trimester and unlike first trimester fatigue, this time you will feel sluggishness because you are not well-rested and are now lugging around 20 odd pounds more. Your growing baby is adding more pressure on major blood vessels making less oxygen available to your brains.

- If you have been exercising, your body will be better equipped to handle the extra weight. However, even the fittest mum can expect to feel the lethargy because of nights of poor sleep. So sleep whenever you can, avoid standing up too quickly, avoid lying on your back when resting and avoid becoming overheated.

Common Concerns

I have my legs waxed. Is this ok during pregnancy?

- There isn't any risk to this procedure. Just be careful not to get overheated while having this done. Your body temperature should not be above 102°F or 39°C for more than 15 minutes.

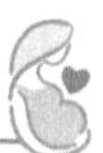

What are the signs of placenta previa and how common is it? Are there things I should avoid if I know I have placenta previa?

- It occurs in about 1: 200 births. The most typical symptom is painless bleeding. It is advisable to avoid intercourse, travel and having a pelvic exam.

What will my doctor do if I have painless bleeding?

- An ultrasound will be ordered to determine the location of the baby. Your doctor will not conduct a pelvic exam as this will cause heavier bleeding and it is recommended that whoever examines you apart from your doctor is informed about your condition.

Intrauterine Fibroids and Pregnancy

- Hormone levels shoot up during pregnancy, causing pre-existing fibroids to grow rapidly. If they degenerate, fibroids can sometimes cause uterine contractions that may result in premature delivery. Often, pregnancies proceed to full term without pain, bleeding or premature delivery. Generally, fibroids do not hurt the developing baby unless they irritate to the point where the uterus starts to contract, triggering premature labor. Unfortunately, there are no sure ways to prevent fibroids from creating problems during pregnancy because when the uterus grows the fibroid wall grows too. The only assurance is, if the fibroid is located far away from the uterine cavity, then the chance for a complicated pregnancy decreases tremendously.

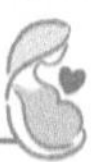

Nutrition

- Your nutritional needs should be met through the foods you eat. But, this is a rather unrealistic demand for most women and therefore necessitates a daily prenatal vitamin dose.

- Some women especially need to depend on these supplements - underweight women, women who had a poor diet prior to conception and women who have multiples. Vegetetarians, poor eaters, those who take certain medications, those tho have an aversion to basics like milk, need these supplements all the more.

- Your doctor is the best judge to decide if you need supplements or if you need more in addition to your prenatal vitamins. Do not take any supplements without your doctor's advice.

- You may find the same old healthy foods boring as you progress further into your pregnancy. To spice up your menu, here are some tips to help you along without the compromise.

- Green leafy vegetables such as spinach and broccoli contain nutrients that are different from the orange group of vegetables such as carrots and beetroot. Include both categories in your diet every day.

- Fruits and vegetables are good any time and are nutritious too. They are high in vitamins and minerals and low in calories - just what you need.

- To control your sweet tooth, set yourself a limit – eg. 100 calories of chocolate a day. Read product labels for a better idea.

- For your salads, different type of lettuce have different nutrients to offer. The darker, the better.

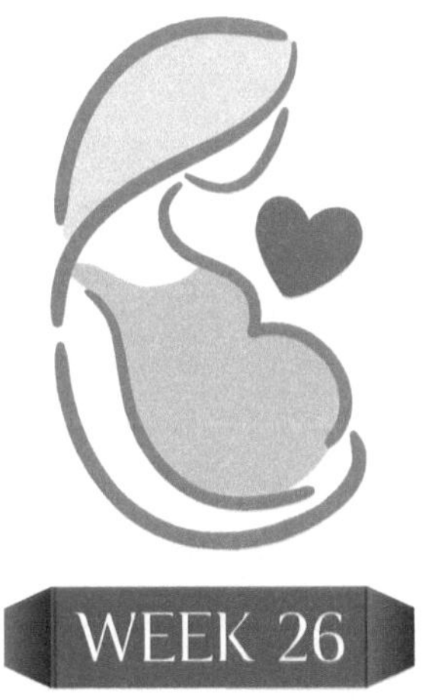

WEEK 26

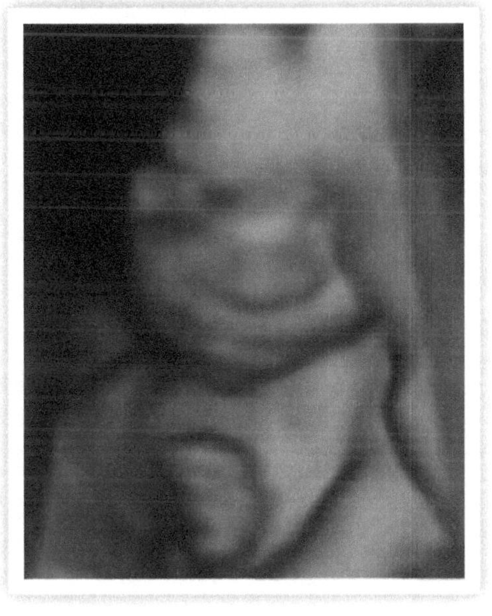

FOETUS AGE 24 WEEKS

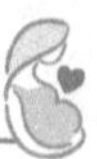

Changes in Baby

- From crown to rump, your baby measures at 9½ inches and weighs about 1½-2 pounds.

- Your baby's eyelashes and eyebrows are well formed now.

- Your baby still looks red and wrinkled, but more fat is collecting under the skin with each passing day. Soon enough, this wrinkly suit will not look wrinkly anymore.

- All the components that make up the eyes have developed, but baby's eyes won't probably open for another 2 weeks.

- This week marks a major milestone in hearing and vision. Your baby's hearing is completely formed and in a couple of weeks, baby will become more sensitive to sound.

- The substance surfactant which keeps the lung tissue from sticking together will be secreted by the air sacs forming in the lungs.

Changes in You

- Progesterone is continuing to slow the movement of food through your digestive tract; your expanding uterus is crowding and pressing on your intestines - the likely consequence is either heartburn or constipation, or both.

- The ligaments supporting your pelvic bones are continuing to become more elastic this month in preparation for childbirth; however these lax muscles give rise to back strain.

- Sleeping is definitely becoming an issue - try sleeping on your left side more often.

- Between now and the next three weeks, you may be tested for gestational diabetes with a glucose tolerance test.

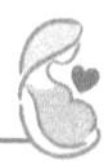

- Sometimes, you probably wish you could take a break from your pregnancy!

Good To Know

Miscellaneous

- All babies have blue eyes in the uterus irrespective of their genes. A baby's eyes don't get the final color until a few months after the birth.

- As your baby grows, your center of gravity will change causing a pregnant woman to be prone to tripping and falling. Hang on to those handrails on the way up and down the stairs.

- Relaxin, the hormone which relaxes the pelvic girdle and softens the cervix is probably named because of this. Its general presence has caused the ligaments, including your feet ligaments to expand. Many women may go up an entire shoe size by the time they deliver. And this change is most likely permanent.

Strep B (Group B streptococcus)

- If a swab were carried out to check for vaginal infection such as thrush, the results may come back positive for Group B strep too. A common infection, it can be dangerous for newborn babies. You will be given an antibiotic IV during labor to prevent the infection from spreading to the baby.

What is Diastasis Recti

- Diastasis Recti refers to the visible separation or gap between your left and right recti muscles. Once again it is due to the hormones that surface during pregnancy, mainly relaxin. Many women are not even aware that they have it.

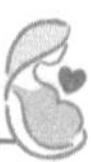

- After delivery, most women will have a gap between the two stomach muscles, known as the rectus muscles. Rectus muscles run vertically down to the pelvis. They may separate in the middle. This separation is termed as diastasis recti and is a type of hernia.

Wholesome Advice

- By now, high heels may not be the wisest choice for you with all that weight gained.

- Fear of labor is universal. Understanding that fear of the unknown is greater than the actual pain is a belief you should hold on to. Labor though intense, doesn't usually start all of a sudden. The contractions usually start erratically and gradually assume more intense proportions. With time, the contractions will become more regular and intense. Though scary, you will handle these painful contractions with or without pain relief. That is the way mother nature intended.

Your Actions Can Impact Your Baby's Growth

Your Wardrobe

- Now is definitely the time to organize your closet if you haven't done so already. In fact it is long overdue! Time to pack away your pre-pregnancy clothes and lingerie (which don't fit anyway) and make room for maternity wear which will be of use for a few months post-partum.

Good buys

- As you grow larger; pants, capris and jeans with tummy panels may become more comfortable.

- Comfortable cotton bras that convert into nursing bras

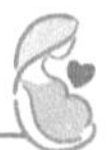

should be good. For the large-breasted, look for supportive wide straps. Buy two bras max at a time because of your changing size.

* Maternity dresses with strings in the back to loosen or tighten the fit.

* Button down shirts long enough to cover your pants panels.

* Flat-soled shoes or slip-on sandals.

Bad buys

* Non-maternity tops that will fit your stomach but will hang badly everywhere else.

* Thong style underwear that make you look sexy but can cause UTI.

* Bras made of synthetic fabrics which can give you skin problems such as nipple irritation or skin rash.

* Wide legged pants which make you look broad all over.

* Over the stomach underwear which tends to be too big for postpartum wear.

Common Concerns

Can I still go for my aerobics lessons?

* Stick to low impact exercises; this means, avoid high kicks to minimize the stress on the pelvic joints and floor muscles. Continue these exercises until the final months when you will need to slow down.

Why is walking good during pregnancy?

* Walking keeps you fit without aching your knees and ankles. It can be done throughout your nine months and

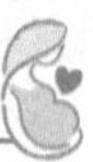

one of the easiest forms of exercise for the non-exercising mom-to-be. If you were fairly inactive before becoming pregnant, start with a slow walk and build this up to brisk walking routines of 20-30 minutes. Alternate the pace with few minutes of brisk walking and then slow walking. As you grow bigger, you may start to walk with short steps and a clumsy swaying motion; pay attention to your gait and posture. Swing your arms for balance, to stabilize your pelvis and intensify your workout.

Nutrition

- Eating fish is healthy and especially good during pregnancy. Women who consume a variety of fish end up having full term babies and babies with higher birth weights. This is important because the longer the baby remains in the womb, the stronger and healthier it will be during delivery.

- Omega-3 fatty acids found in fish is responsible for preventing premature births; it triggers a hormone which helps prevent pregnancy induced hypertension and preeclampsia as well.

- Fish is the right choice of protein because it is safe, low in fat and high in vitamin B, iron, zinc, selenium and copper. Eating most varieties on a frequent basis should be no problem.

- If you are a vegetarian or simply dislike fish, add canola oil, flaxseed, soybeans, walnuts and wheat germ to your diet plan because of the linolenic oil content, a type of omega-3 fatty acid found in them. Some research indicates eating fatty fish or fish oil capsules may also enhance your baby's intellect since fish oil is important

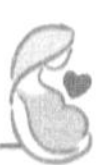

for fetal brain development. While it is good to include omega-3 in your food plan, do not exceed 2.4g of omega 3 per day. Not all fish are safe for eating. Some fish are contaminated with dangerous substances derived from man-made pollutants called methyl mercury.

- Methyl mercury can pass from mother to baby giving rise to neurological problems. Babies are especially vulnerable because of the rapid brain development that takes place inside the uterus. Pregnant women and those trying to conceive should be cautioned from taking certain types of fish more than once a month. These include shark, swordfish and tuna (fresh or frozen). Nursing mothers should limit those fish to once a week. Canned tuna is safer but don't exceed more than 6 oz per week. Avoid all raw fish during pregnancy including sushi. If you are not sure about what to avoid, seek expert advice of a dietician.

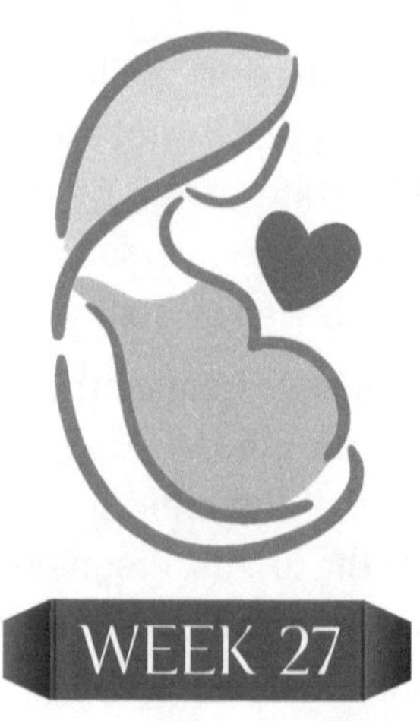

WEEK 27

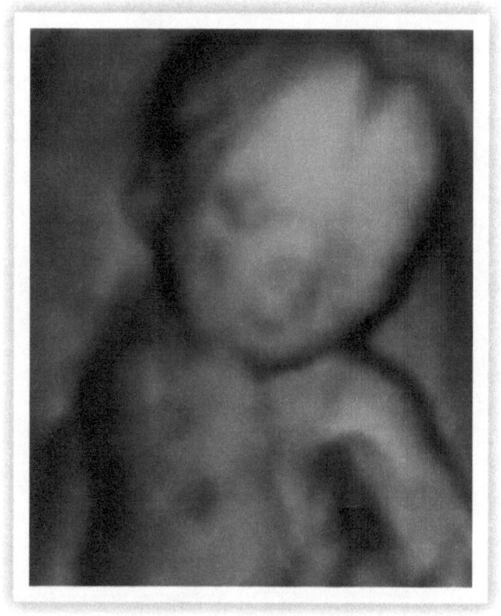

FOETUS AGE 25 WEEKS

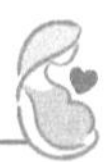

Changes in Baby

* From crown to rump, your baby measures at 9½ inches and weighs about 2 pounds.

* By now, your baby will resemble a thinner, smaller, redder version of what it will look like at birth.

* Lungs, liver and immune system aren't fully mature yet.

* Baby is starting to distinguish your voice from the rest, although it is rather difficult to hear clearly through the thick vernix covering the ears and through the amniotic fluid in the uterus.

* For most babies the most active period is between weeks 27 and 32.

Changes in You

* You are probably gaining weight at a steady pace and may be aware that you are starting to feel more tired.

* Shooting pain caused by baby's weight can be discomforting. Termed sciatica; walking, bending and lifting further aggravates this condition. Warm baths, ice packs may help.

* Since the amniotic fluid is lowered by half, you will be able to see bony knees and elbows poking out whenever your baby kicks and turns.

* Stretch marks on your breasts and abdomen become more pronounced.

* Your heart rate may have increased causing you to feel flushed with little exertion.

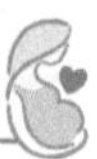

Good to Know

Miscellaneous

- Babies have more taste buds at birth than they will have later in life.

- If you are flying and have a big belly, you need your doctor's note of approval to get on a plane. Some airlines do not allow travel after week 32 or as late as within 30 days of your due date without your doctor's note.

- Endorphins, the happy hormone, helps numb the pain and stress of childbirth. After birth, on the same day, this hormone drops sharply. Endorphins can be increased with exercise.

Cholesterol

- Your cholesterol level may rise. Cholesterol is used by you and your baby's placenta to manufacture progesterone. This hormone is responsible for preventing pre-term birth, helping maintain cell's oxygen levels and regulating metabolism.

Breech baby

- A breech presentation is quite common in the early months of pregnancy as there is plenty of room for the fetus to swim around. A very good percentage of babies are present in the normal head down position (vertex) at the onset of labor. However, about 3 to 4 percent of babies remain in breech positions, with the head up toward the mother's ribs instead of down at week 40. That would mean the feet or buttocks will have to be delivered first.

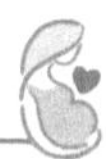

Wholesome Advice

* Knowing your options for pain relief often eases anxiety. There is medication if you need it.
* Be open with your partner and your doctor about your fears. Becoming informed about the process and obtaining information from medical professionals will help ease your fears.
* Having other children makes it hard for pregnant women to set their priorities straight and take good care of themselves. Let some work and chores go and have your partner pitch in.

Your Actions Can Impact Your Baby's Growth

Calf stretch

* If you are bothered by leg cramps at night, a good exercise before going to bed is the calf stretch.
  * Lean one side of your body against a wall. Reach one leg out behind you, keeping your heel on the floor.
  * Lean into the wall to increase the stretch of your calf.
  * Hold for 20-30 seconds then repeat with the other leg.

If you don't work out...

* Some of us are not the type to work out or visit the gym daily. If that is the case, figure out what it is that will keep you going - you don't have to pump iron or ride the stationary bike. Sweeping and mopping the floors of your house can be equivalent to some minutes on a treadmill (depending on the size of your house). Vacuuming for 15-20 minutes, walking to the local store are great ways to exercise without having to actually 'work out'.

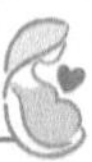

Going up the scales

- If you are gaining weight a little too fast and need to slow down or if your doctor recommends that you cut back, first stop looking at your weight and worrying. Then cut down on your fat intake - this is the only nutritional requirement that is safe to restrict. So no butter on your toast, no oil and rich salad dressings on your salad and avoid fried foods altogether.

Common Concerns

Why do I keep gaining weight with each baby?

- Your body undergoes additional changes with each subsequent pregnancy. There is tendency to gain a few pounds with each baby. The weight gain is not a permanent fixture if you are careful about your diet. Stay away from nutritional losers like sugars and fats. Another reason is pregnant women with other children tend to be too busy to take care of themselves and tend to take meals on the run. You need to allow time to pay attention to what you eat and make time for a simple exercise like brisk walking. A good intake of fruit and vegetables and other healthy foods will minimize the weight gain and keep you healthy.

What about non-ionizing radiation?

- Current research confirms that non-ionizing radiation that is emitted by microwave ovens, TVs and computers isn't harmful. Still, preventive steps to take are: sitting at least 1.25 meters from your computer; not to stand in front of your microwave when heating food; and sitting at least 3 meters from the front of the TV screen. This applies to when you are not pregnant as well.

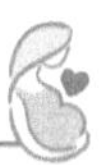

Nutrition

- Some important vitamins that will help you through your pregnancy are vitamins A, B & E. Vitamin A is essential to human reproduction. Deficiency in this vitamin is not so much an issue as an excessive intake is.

- Retinol derived from fish oils is a concern when taken in excess; the beta-carotene form obtained from plant life is safe. The recommended dose is 2700 IU for women of child bearing age with a maximum dose at 5000 IU.

- Supplements are not usually necessary as the foods you eat provide an adequate supply of vitamin A. Read food labels to get an idea of vitamin A content. B vitamins are important during pregnancy and they include B6, folic acid and B12. They play a crucial role in the development of your baby's nerves and formation of blood cells.

- Lack of B12 leads to anemia in the mother. Good food sources of this group of vitamins are milk, eggs, bananas, potatoes, brown rice, etc.

- Vitamin E is important as it helps in fat metabolism and building of muscles and red blood cells. If you are a meat eater, your vitamin E dose is taken care of through your meals.

- Pregnant women who are vegetarians or those who are meat intolerant for some reason have a harder time getting their vitamin E dose. Vegetarian foods rich in this vitamin are olive oil, wheat germ, spinach and dried fruits.

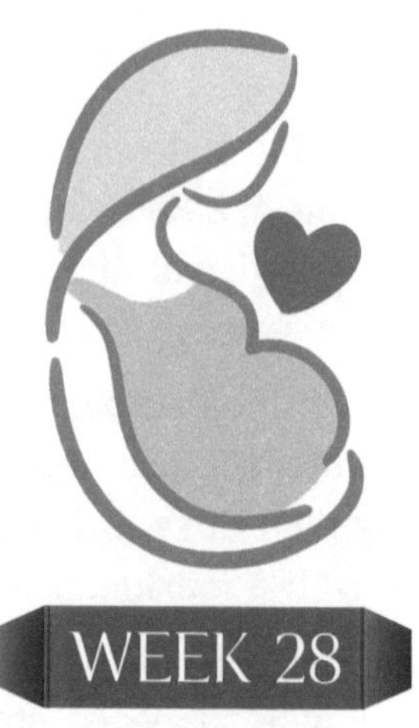

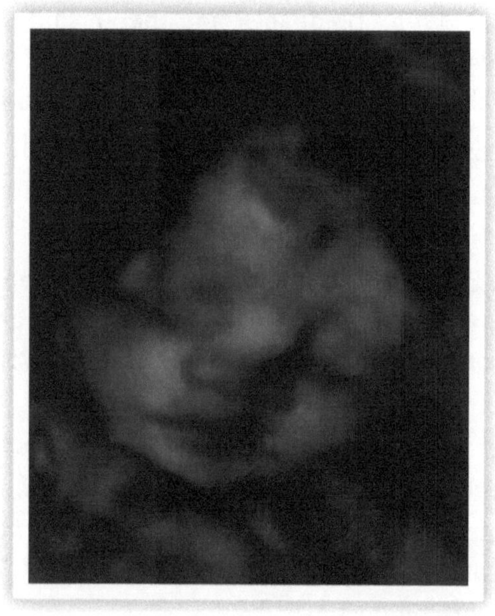

FOETUS AGE 26 WEEKS

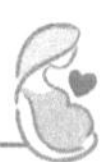

Changes in Baby

- From crown to rump, your baby measures at 10 inches and weighs about 2.3 pounds or 1kg.
- Baby's head is more in proportion with it's body now.
- If baby is a boy, his testes are descending.
- The placenta receives about 400 ml of blood from the mother's circulation every minute.
- Baby's skin is still wrinkled but fat is continuing to develop underneath.
- Baby is developing the ability to orientate itself within its space.
- Baby responds to stimuli including pain, light and sound.
- Your baby's lungs are now capable of breathing air.
- Your baby's eyes are capable of opening this week.

Changes in You

- By the end of this week you would have completed 70% of your pregnancy.
- You are gaining more weight.
- From now you, will be seeing your doctor every 2 weeks then weekly from week 36.
- Your perspiration can get trapped in the skin folds which can be irritating. Try using talcum powder.
- If you are going to get stretch marks, you probably have them by now.

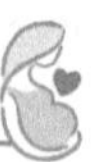

Good to Know

Term Baby

- Why doesn't pregnancy end at week 37 since it is considered full term? The reason is that although baby is considered fully developed and it can survive outside the uterus, baby still needs more time to add weight and develop its lungs and immune system further.

Issues on labor you can check beforehand:

- Labor and delivery are not in your control. It makes sense to check with your doctor on key issues and be emotionally prepared for the consequences.

- Shaving: more and more doctors do not require that you be shaved, although in some instances, if you have a c-section (caesarean) you may be shaved.

- Induction after waters break: many doctors consider it routine to induce within 24 hours of rupture for fear of infection.

- Fetal monitoring: some women prefer no restrictions in movement during active labor but with constant fetal monitoring this is not possible.

- Food: most doctors prefer an empty stomach because digestion doesn't work well during labor.

Wholesome Advice

Put yourself as your first concern and don't feel guilty.

- Pamper yourself - you deserve it!

- Stay positive despite what you are going through. List all the things you are looking forward to about your baby's arrival.

- Good buys, if you are looking for ways to lift your spirits, are earrings, scarves, necklaces and a great haircut.

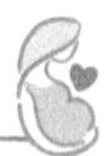

- Remember that hot weather, standing for long periods or low blood sugar can make you feel dizzy and prone to fainting. Drink water and stay in shaded areas.

Your Actions Can Impact Your Baby's Growth

Low Fat ≠ Low Taste

If you are trying to put a halt to your weight gain, here are some ideas you can use:

- Cook in a non-stick pan and use water to keep your food from sticking.

- Grill meats instead of frying them.

- Roast meats on a raised rack so that the juices drip into the pan.

- Reduce the fat in salad dressing by replacing half of the oil with water.

- For creamy dressings, use yoghurt or cottage cheese instead of sour cream or mayo.

Body temperature

- If your hands turn clammy or you get hot or cold flashes, your body is messaging you that it is having a hard time regulating the internal thermometer. Your baby faces the risk of getting overheated just as you do and blood flowing to the uterus will be diverted to the skin as the body tries to cool itself off. Your temperature should be less than 38.3°C or 101°F (when taken under the arm) after exercising. Keep a close watch on this.

Just how much of exercise?

- Exercise too little and not much is achieved; exercise too much and you may harm yourself. A full workout for a

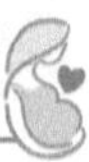

pregnant woman on a regular basis should last about 30-60 minutes, from warm up to cool down. Further, your heart rate should not be over 140 for more than 15 minutes, although this again depends on your health and your exercise history.

Common Concerns

What does having protein in the urine mean?

* The presence of protein in your urine informs how your kidneys are performing. Small amounts are not uncommon and simply mean your kidneys are working harder during this time. Your body is fighting a minor infection and your urine sample will be sent for analysis to determine whether you have a urine infection. Antibiotics may be prescribed and in your following appointment the protein level will be checked, to check for changes. If there are high levels of protein present, a blood sample may be taken to check for preeclampsia.

Will I have any more ultrasound scans?

* You are unlikely to need an ultrasound scan in late pregnancy unless yours is a multiple pregnancy, your previous baby was small or you have a health complication such as hypertension or diabetes etc. A scan can be advised if your baby's position is unclear or if there is some concern over how the baby is thriving or to measure your amniotic level. If you have a low lying placenta, expect to be scanned again at week 36.

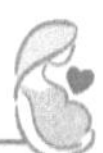

Nutrition

- Certain foods you should eliminate altogether and some you should make it a point to include are outlined below.

Food to Eat	Daily Serving
Dark green, dark yellow fruits & vegetables	1
Fruits & vegetables with Vitamin C (tomatoes & citrus fruits)	2
Other fruits and vegetables	2
Bread and cereals (whole grain variety)	4
Dairy products including milk	4
Protein (meat, eggs, fish)	2
Dried beans, peas, nuts, seeds	2
Foods to Eat in Moderation	**Daily Serving**
Caffeine	200 mg
Fat	In limits
Sugar	In limits
Foods to Avoid	
Anything with alcohol, additives	

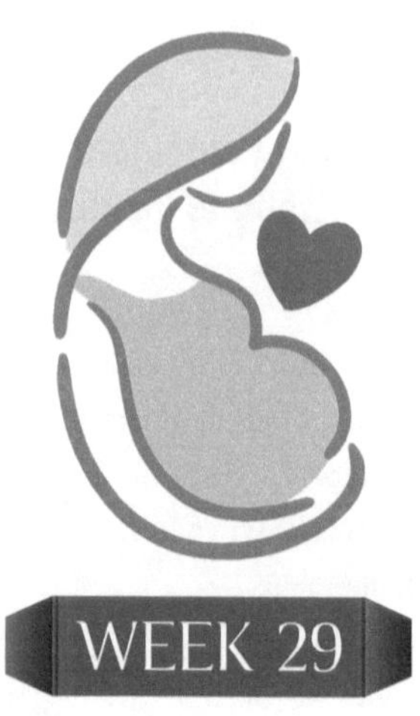

WEEK 29

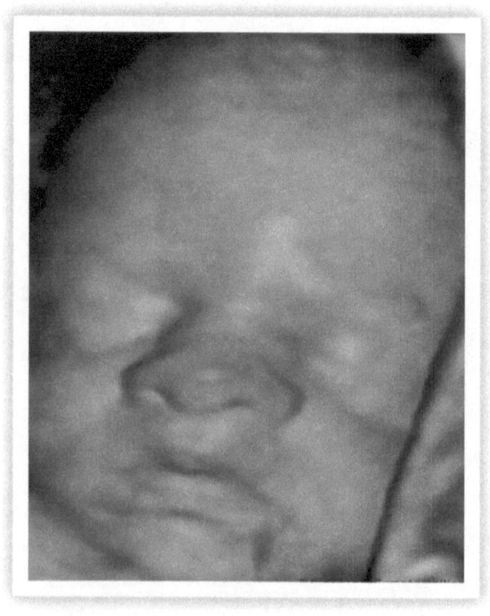

FOETUS AGE 27 WEEKS

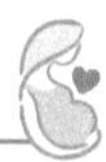

Changes in Baby

* From crown to rump, your baby measures at 10½ inches and weighs about 2.4 pounds or 1.02 kgs.

* Your baby's adrenal glands are producing a chemical which will be made into estriol, a form of estrogen. Estriol is thought to stimulate the production of prolactin by your body which in turn produces milk in the mother. That way, even if your baby arrives early, you will be able to breastfeed.

* Baby is growing eyelashes, adding fat and developing its brain.

* Researchers speculate that due to brain activity, babies can even dream at this time.

Changes in You

* As levels of prolactin increase in your body, your breasts may secrete colostrum.

* Prolactin also has a sedating effect, causing you to nap more often as you did in the first trimester.

* You may notice that your eyelids and face are becoming puffy, especially in the morning. This is because of increased blood circulation.

* Your uterus now exerts pressure on your bladder - frequent trips to the washroom may also remind you of your first trimester.

* The tubes that link your kidney, bladder and urethra are compressed; which means you are not able to empty your bladder efficiently.

* You may also leak urine when you laugh or cough.

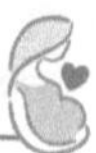

Good to Know

- The extra pound that most pregnant ladies gain this week will be partly fluid.

- Oxytoxin: A synthetic hormone, Oxytoxin, similar to one that your body manufactures naturally can be administered to induce labor. Oxytoxin may be used to augment labor that is already happening. If your labor is taking unusually long to progress or is inadequate, your doctor may use Oxytoxin to move things along. The contractions produced are no stronger and no more painful than contractions that occur naturally during labor.

What is a Doppler Scan?

- Doppler scan is a special scan which uses black and white or colour images to examine the blood flowing through the umbilical cord between the placenta and the baby.

- This non-invasive test differs from the normal ultrasound in which a slightly different sound wave is used which bounces off moving red blood cells and shows the speed rate at which the cells are moving.

- It can be done at the same time as an ultrasound; the same equipment is used to measure the blood flow in various body parts such as the umbilical cord, liver, heart and brain.

Wholesome Advice

- Squatting during delivery opens up your pelvis even wider so the baby has more room to move down into the birth canal. Using the wall for support is a great way to practice. Once you have built up the strength, you can try using a sturdy chair instead of the wall.

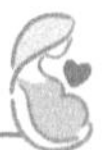

- Regular exercising, especially squatting, swimming and walking can relieve constipation. It is tempting to just sit around, but keeping your body moving slowly which will keep your insides moving as well. Leg cramps can also be prevented with exercise.

- Don't forget to Kegel - it will keep your pelvic floor toned.

Your Actions Can Impact Your Baby's Growth

- *Posture and Meals:* Sit with a good posture when you eat as slouching can put extra pressure on your stomach. To ease heartburn, chew gum or suck on lozenges (not mints) to produce a flow of saliva which may help control stomach acid. Good sitting posture helps ease backache and strengthens those muscles. Avoid lying down or stooping immediately after meals and if you have trouble sitting comfortably, place a pillow behind your back e.g. when driving.

- *Antacids:* Antacids are available over the counter at the pharmacy and do not contain ingredients that can be absorbed and therefore enter your baby's bloodstream. They merely neutralize acid in the esophagus and stomach. Avoid indigestion tablets which are absorbed into the bloodstream. Eating yoghurt and milk can help, but cheese can worsen heartburn.

- *Drinks and Heartburn:* Avoid having a lot to drink with meals if you have heartburn issue. You tend to swallow more air when you drink while you are eating. Avoid caffeine and carbonated drinks. If you feel like having a carbonated drink, try orange juice with soda water or add soda water to any other favorite juice.

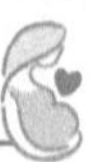

Common Concerns

I have become very clumsy recently - is this normal?

* Yes, this is expected. It is a temporary side effect of pregnancy. You are now carrying more weight, your center of gravity has shifted with your growing uterus and your joints are all loosening due to pregnancy hormones. Tripping and falling is a huge fear, but rest assured your baby is well cushioned in the waters and the bony pelvis provides adequate protection. If you do fall, contact your doctor to be sure that all is ok with you and your baby. Avoid risky situations such as wet or uneven surfaces. If clumsiness is accompanied by dizziness, headaches, blurry vision or pain, contact your doctor at the earliest.

I have become forgetful and this is bothering me

* So much is going on in your head - everything is about to change very soon for you. Preoccupation with issues makes a person forgetful versus a clear headed individual. Carry a small notebook so that you can jot down reminders. Maintain a calendar. Keep items you often use such as your wallet in the same place.

Nutrition

* Depression during pregnancy can occur due to both simple and complex reasons.

* Changes in hormones impacts you at an emotional and physical level and can cause you to feel nausea, exhaustion and mood swings.

* Having a baby involves having a change to your personal circumstances - there is loss of freedom and even a reason for old buried fears and anxieties to reappear.

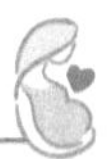

- Symptoms are - negative feelings, mood swings, detachment, disturbed sleep, panic attacks and change in appetite.

- You can include yoga into your schedule; it has proven to be effective in helping you deal with depression. Forms of yoga are many, but they all aim at balancing your mind and body thus leading you to physical relaxation and improved well-being.

- Pay attention to your diet as nutritional deficiencies play a role by causing your hormones to go out of whack. Zinc deficiency is most common during pregnancy; eat zinc-rich foods such as eggs, sunflower seeds and whole-meal bread.

- Also boost your intake of vitamin C and B complex.

- Avoid sugary foods and stimulants such as caffeine and alcohol which have an adverse effect on mood.

- Discuss your feelings with a counselor or friend.

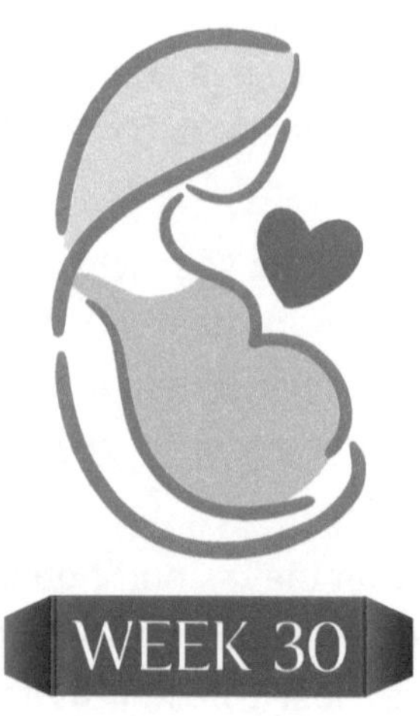

WEEK 30

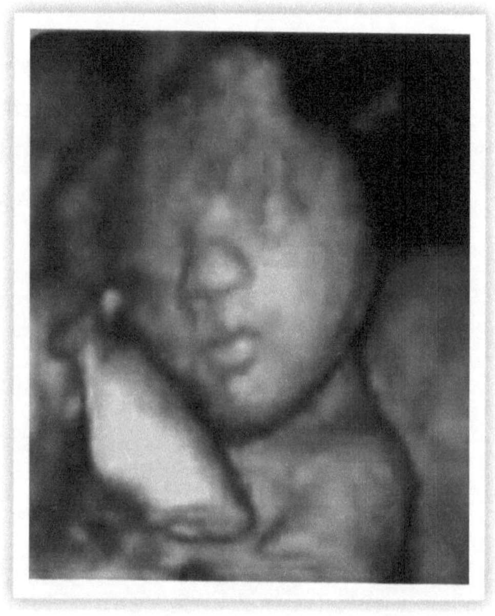

FOETUS AGE 28 WEEKS

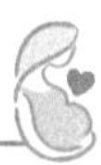

Changes in Baby

- From crown to rump, your baby almost measures at 11 inches and weighs about 2½-3 pounds.
- Your baby is now probably lying in a curled-up position.
- Movements are less; most babies adopt a head-down position. If your baby is one of those who is in breech or lying sideways, there are still 6 weeks for baby to change to head-down or cephalic position for birth.
- Baby will only gain a few inches in length from now till delivery.
- The most important organ, the brain, continues to develop at a rapid pace.
- Baby is still floating in about 1½ pints of fluid, ample room for movement.

Changes in You

- You have now been officially pregnant for 7 months.
- You are big now - your belly is the size of a watermelon.
- You may feel your heart pounding or have shortness of breath when you exert.
- Your abdominal muscles have loosened so when you are lying down you can't get up as quickly as before. Roll to one side before getting up.
- You may have started the pregnancy 'waddle'.

Fetal Movements in the Third Trimester

- Fetal movements in the third trimester will not be same as those felt in the earlier months. Then, the uterus was roomier to accommodate your baby's kicking and punching and other acrobatics. Now, conditions are

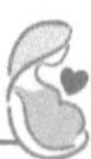

getting too cramped for baby's gymnastics. All mothers and babies are different, and one pregnancy is different from another, so the amount of fetal movement in the third trimester is bound to be different as well.

Good to Know

* Swelling in your legs and feet are normal and common unless it involves your hand and face.

Baby Gadgets

* Babies change weekly on what they like and don't like. So don't give up on baby gadgets.

* Babies love to swing. With proper supervision, baby swings are appropriate from birth to about 9 months or a weight of 25 lbs or 11.3 kg. The back and forth motion soothes a crying baby and helps a newborn fall asleep. Colicky babies benefits from this movement too.

* Invest in a good stroller with a built-in infant car seat. You will need the infant car seat whenever you go out with your baby. This 2-in-1 is convenient - just pop them from the carrier in the stroller to the car. Babies sleep comfortably in a car seat rather than their cribs. The car seat can also be used to soothe your baby by gently rocking it back and forth.

What is Chorioamnionitis?

* One in 100 pregnant women are diagnosed with chorioamnionitis, which is a serious infection of the amniotic fluid, fetal membranes and placental tissues. Chorioamnionitis is regarded as a major cause of preterm premature rupture of membranes (PPROM) and premature labor.

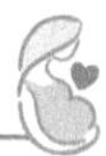

Wholesome Advice

- Start building on your baby's library now with board books. You can start reading to your baby when it is few months old.

- There are many 'must-have baby items' that you can get confused. The bottom line is you don't really need most of them. All you need right away, besides the basics – diapers, onesies and blankets - are a car seat and a bassinette.

Your Actions Can Impact Your Baby's Growth

Elevate your legs and feet

- A 10-15 minutes break, spent lying down on your back with both your feet and legs elevated does wonders for you during your final trimester. This position will boost the circulation in your legs and give your back the much needed rest it needs. This tip is useful not just at the end of the day but at any time when you can squeeze a quick break.

The non-drug approach for depression

- Depression is a disease that can be treated and controlled. The most common treatment for depression comes in pill form, which may not be a wise option right now. There are non-drug treatments that may work for you for minor symptoms of depression. If you are on medication (approved by your doctor) these steps can help your medication work even better.

- _Magnesium:_ Make sure you get enough of this mineral found in fruits, nuts and vegetables and omega fatty acids found in fish and olive oil.

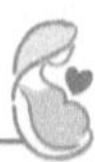

- *Low carbs:* Avoid sugar and processed carbs.

- *Moderate exercise:* Exercise helps to alter negative feelings from escalating. Moderate exercise such as walking, yoga and swimming for half an hour a day makes your body release more endorphins which elevates your spirits.

- *Balanced blood sugar:* Keep food in your stomach at all times and drink plenty of water. Low blood sugar is known to increase feelings of depression and irritability.

- *Control stress:* Avoid stress if you can - now is not a good time to take on new responsibilities if you can avoid them.

- *Avoid self-medication:* However bad it may be, don't use alcohol, smoking or drugs as a way out. Seek safe alternatives.

Common Concerns

Is it normal to feel stressed?

- Lots of pregnant women suffer from stress. Your mind maybe crowded by all kinds of thoughts including your unborn baby's health, your upcoming labor; you may wonder about how you will manage the labor and the aftermath, whether you have bought everything. It is however important to de-stress and not let worry consume you.

Will stress harm my unborn baby?

- Isolated stress experience from time to time will have no harmful impact on you or your baby. However, prolonged stress, especially in the early part of pregnancy can increase your chances of pregnancy complications such as preeclampsia and premature birth and there seems to be link to hyperactive disorders in pre-school children.

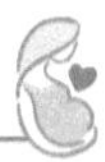

If you are undergoing unmanageable stress it is important to seek help.

Is there anything we can do to prepare for caring for our newborn?

- Read parenting books of journals together. Discuss issues that are raised such as baby safety, breast feeding vs bottle feeding. Reading gives the couple something to do together, besides the useful information. Discuss any plans of action you might have with regards to roles and duties and external help you may need once the baby arrives.

Nutrition
- Constipation is a common concern during pregnancy and is caused by a slowdown in bowel movement due to the hormone progesterone. Constipation or pressure from the uterus may lead to swollen veins or hemorrhoids. Vein problem in legs is caused by the increased weight and blood volume. To remedy the situation or even prevent them, eat foods that are rich in vitamin C and bioflavonoids such as garlic, onions and parsley. The following tips will help ease constipation:
  - Drink plenty of water
  - Limit processed food
  - Eat plenty of fiber rich foods
  - Eat psyllium seeds to soften stools
  - Eat oat bran, dried fruits, papayas, figs and peas
  - Eat almonds and bananas for bulk and honey for lubrication

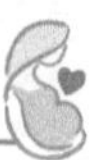

- 2-3 helpings of salad a day will provide plenty of useful fiber

Water

- Drinking water during pregnancy is one of the most important ways you can offer protection to your unborn child because adequate hydration prevents premature labor. Dehydration can cause uterine contractions leading to premature birth.

- UTI is more commonplace because of the hormonal changes your body undergoes. Again, this can cause premature labor to kick in.

- During pregnancy, your metabolism revs up. Before your blood volume increases, adequate fluids help dissipate some of this additional heat.

- Hormonal changes can cause constipation; drinking water improves regularity.

- Staying hydrated keeps headaches, dry skin and complexion problems at bay.

- Aim for at least 8 glasses of water per day. One easy way is to keep water within easy reach at all times. Experiment which taste or temperature suits your taste buds best; icy cold or room temperature or mixed with some flavour for those who don't like it bland. When considering fluids, don't include colas or fizzy drinks or even fruit juices. Soft drinks and carbonated beverages leave you bloated and full. Fruit juices contain sugar; don't go overboard. Coffee and tea contain caffeine. So stick with water.

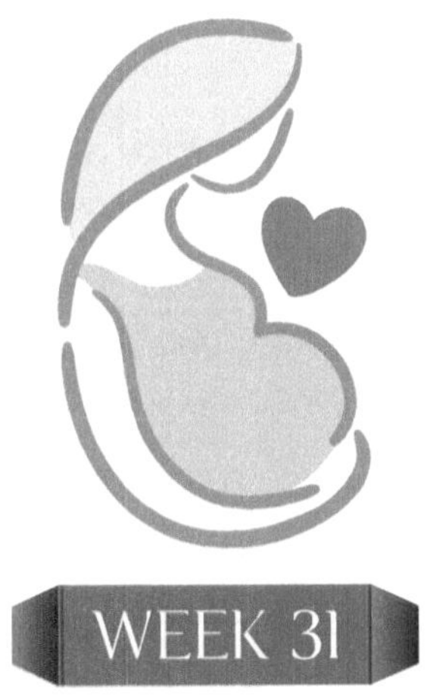

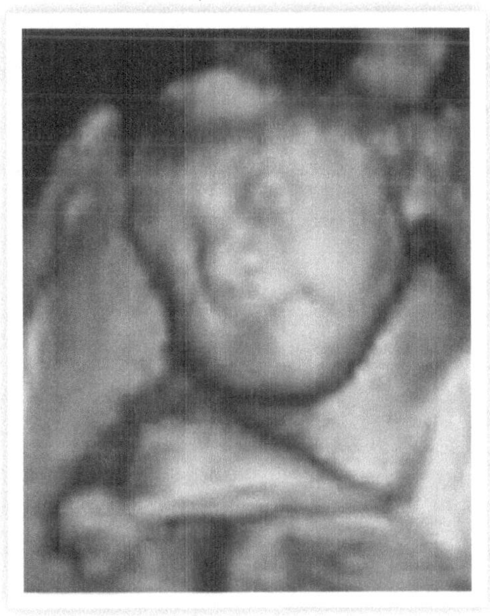

FOETUS AGE 29 WEEKS

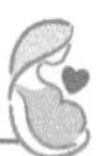

Changes in Baby

- From crown to rump, your baby almost measures at 11¼ inches and weighs about 2½-3½ pounds.
- Your baby begins to run out of room as it gains weight. About 10 kicks an hour can be felt. Baby's kicks and movements can be more intensely felt now.
- Both the lanugo and vernix begin to disappear.
- Your baby starts to grow plumper and its skin begins to fill out and become smoother.

Changes in You

- With heavier breasts, start wearing a well-fitting bra night and day - good support will make you feel more comfortable.
- The extra inches and shift in gravity can make you more clumsy and prone to falls and knocks.
- Puffy face and limbs are considered normal if you do not have protein in your urine and your blood pressure is normal.

Good to Know

- According to scientists, music does have a calming effect on babies. Music mixed with womb sounds are the best – the whooshing blood and mother's heartbeat soothes fussy babies.

Myths about predicting baby's gender

- Ultrasound can always predict the baby's sex.
- If the woman is on top when the baby is conceived, it's a boy.

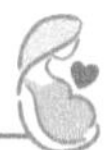

- If a pregnant woman gains weight in the face, it's a girl baby.

- A round belly means the baby is a girl.

- A moody pregnant woman means she is carrying a girl child.

- If the fetal heart rate is fast, means the baby is a girl.

- If a lock dangled over a pregnant belly swings back and forth, the baby is a boy.

What is Nonstress Test?

- Nonstress test is a simple, painless procedure in which a baby's heartbeat is continuously monitored for 20 minutes or more and the details are recorded for evaluation. The logic behind the test is, that like adults, a baby's heartbeat should accelerate when it is active i.e. moving and kicking. The nonstress test can be done whenever the need arises, so there is no specific time for it.

The procedure itself...

- You will be made to lie down on your left side. Two electronic devices will be strapped to your belly.

- The transducer ultrasound will monitor baby's heartbeat.

- The other device will record any uterine contractions felt by the mother.

- If there are no movements, the technician may wake baby up with a buzzer.

- The test takes about 20 minutes to an hour.

- It will be sensible to pee and tuck in a snack before the procedure as the whole thing can last for an hour.

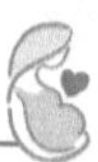

Wholesome Advice

* Try sitting cross legged when you can. Remember to keep your back straight.

* There are several situations where you may be prescribed bed rest, such as pregnancy induced hypertension, preeclampsia, or pre-term labor. Find out from your doctor on all there is to know if you have to be in such a situation.

Your Actions Can Impact Your Baby's Growth

If you have Diarrhea

* During pregnancy your body is more reactive to toxins in foods and does its best to expel food as quickly as possible to keep harmful stuff out.

* Mild diarrhea is nothing to worry about - it should go away after the offending stuff has been expelled.

* Food poisoning and serious cramps and diarrhea can be dangerous, because they cause your body to lose precious fluids bringing about electrolyte imbalance in your system. Your body is robbed of valuable nutrients.

* In the worst case scenario dehydration can cause the mother to have premature contractions.

* If diarrhea doesn't go away after 24 hours, contact your doctor. If you feel cramping and abdominal pain that you feel is not gas related, alert your doctor.

The Gassy and Bloated Feeling

* With pregnancy, your digestive tract tends to slow down to allow your body to absorb as much nutrition from your food.

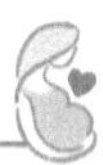

- Your stomach enzymes take its own time to process whatever you eat.

- This slowdown causes you to burp more, feel bloated and gassy.

- It is important to know what foods are causing you the problem; milk products can be a problem if you are lactose intolerant. Certain vegetables are gassier than others. Eliminate or reduce its intake and seek other substitutes to balance things out.

- As your pregnancy advances, your growing uterus will put pressure on your stomach which will further slow down digestion making you feel more bloated and gassy.

- Check with your doctor on what OTC medications are safe to take.

- If your gassy feeling is more akin to abdominal pain or cramping or if there is blood in your stool, severe diarrhea or constipation or excess vomiting, call your doctor right away.

Common Concern

Will my lack of sleep harm my baby?

- Your baby can sleep when you are wide awake; your baby sleeps independently of you. Babies aren't bothered by the same sounds that keep their mothers awake - layers of skin and muscles and the amniotic fluid keeps baby insulated from external sounds and disturbances.

- However, that doesn't mean that baby is cut off from the outside world. Loud sounds or sudden jerks can wake it and the mother may feel a sudden punch or kick as a result.

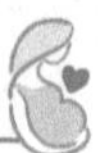

- Your baby's health is at risk if your lack of sleep affects your ability to function e.g. exhaustion causing the mother to suddenly fall.

Nutrition

- Your blood volume is still increasing, so you need to be good with your iron and vitamin C intake.

- Your weight gain is higher now than at any other time of your pregnancy. Your body is preparing itself for breast-feeding.

- It is important to take in the right kind of fat i.e. polyunsaturated - to obtain the essential fatty acids. Baby's brain is growing faster than ever. The brain cells are increasing at a rate of 100,000 cells a minute! 70% of the calories your baby receives are used for brain growth.

- When your baby is born, its brain weighs about 350g of which 60% is fat (20% of this is a long chain of poly-unsaturated fatty acids or LCPs).

- There is evidence that DHA (an active form of Omega 3) helps prevent pregnancy induced hypertension, reduces the likelihood of premature birth, increases a baby's birth weight, improves its IQ, visual and cognitive brain functions and protects against heart disease.

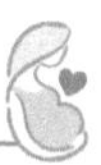

Nutrient	For Mother	For Baby
Vitamin A: A powerful antioxidant	For production of hormones for lactation and good immunity	For maintaining healthy mucous membranes
B Vitamins: Needed in increased amounts	B1 for energy production, B6 for protein metabolism, folate to make DNA and B12 to make red blood cells	B1 for energy production
Vitamin E: A powerful antioxidant	Speeds up wound healing, increases skin suppleness, may strengthen uterine muscles	For development of nervous system and heart
Vitamins C, K: Developed naturally in the gut, but not in the baby's gut so may be given orally at birth	Vit. C for iron absorption, hormone production and resistance to infection. Vit. K for blood clotting	Vit. K for blood clotting
Calcium: Fetus takes up at a rate of 350mg a day	For prevention of preeclampsia and raised BP; (with vitamin D to ease labor pains)	For development of bones and teeth
Zinc: Boys take 5 times as much zinc as girls; deficiency is also linked to undescended testicles	For hormonal balance; may help prevent stretch marks	For development and growth of reproductive system
Other minerals, Iron: Intake must be kept high because it takes 6 weeks to build supplies	Iron for manufacture of red blood cells (vitamins C, B6, B12 and folate improve absorption)	Selenium for brain development, phosphorus for bone development

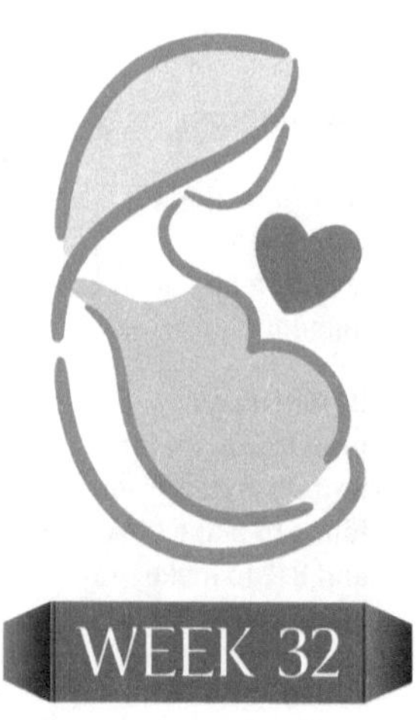

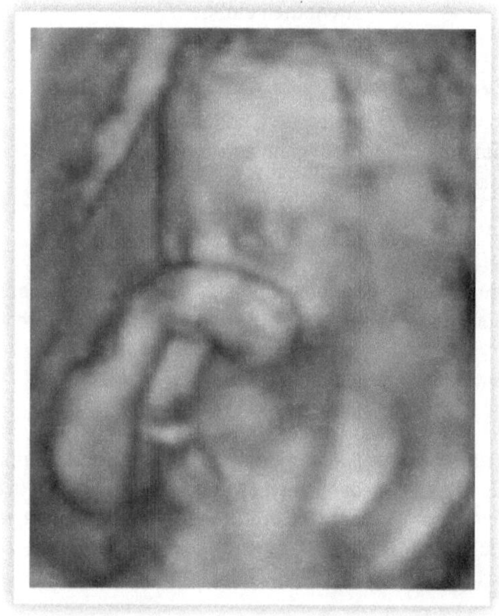

FOETUS AGE 30 WEEKS

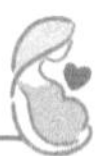

Changes in Baby

- From head to toe, your baby almost measures at 18 inches, and weighs about 4 pounds.

- Baby's foot or other body parts can be felt around your ribcage from time to time. That's because baby is running out of room.

- Baby's kicks and movements may seem more muted now because of the shortage of space.

Changes in You

- You are probably running out of patience!

- You may experience shooting pains down your legs during the day and bad leg cramps at night.

- Many women go through fatigue and PMS like symptoms.

- Sleeping comfortably is getting more and more difficult.

- You are gaining about a pound a week and about a half of that goes to your baby.

- Due to increased blood circulation, your eyelids and face are becoming puffy mostly in the mornings.

Good to Know

- *Sex matters:* The bigger you get belly wise the harder it can be to have sex. If your baby drops early, penetration may be unpleasant and even painful.

- Another impediment to sex in the third trimester is your aching back.

- Miscellaneous: Dilation is measured in centimeters with the cervix opening from 0-10 cms or 4 inches during labor. Dilation is good for your doctor when the opening of the cervix is examined during a pelvic exam.

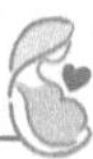

Wholesome Advice

* You may want to invest in some proper maternity support underwear or a maternity belt specially designed to give you the much needed back and belly support. Maternity belts are designed to fit right under your belly and are expandable.

* If you are too busy to eat proper meals, don't be tempted to fill up on empty calories. Ideally you should eat regular meals, but when that's not possible, fill up on fresh or dried fruit, energy bars and yoghurt. Stock up these snacks in your desk drawer if you are working.

* Take calcium supplements with food to aid absorption of the mineral.

Your Actions Can Impact Your Baby's Growth

* Hidden fats are something you should be concerned about if you eat out often or are gaining too much weight.

* Words to look out for include pan-fried, crispy fried, creamed, buttery, au-gratin, etc.

* Instead choose grilled, baked or steamed foods from the menu or check with the waiter if 'good' fat like olive oil can be used or if the oil and other fatty ingredients can be omitted when your dish is being prepared.

* *Walking:* Walking, like swimming or yoga is good in the final trimester. If you don't have time for work out, walking can be easily built into your daily routine.

* Keep up your walking routine for as long as you can (this can come handy when you go into labor) but avoid paths and trails that can throw you off balance.

* As you move closer to your due date, you may feel safer

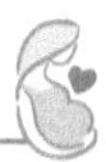

walking a closer distance to your home or your car in case of any emergency.

Common Concern

Does labor hurt the baby?

* Although the route from the uterus to the outside world is relative short, it can be a challenging journey. Your baby is squeezed and pushed down the vaginal canal during the toughest phase of labor. The bony passageway of the mother's pelvis makes it harder as well. As such, baby's heartbeat slows down in intervals during the journey, but it is expected and not a cause for concern.

Why do I snore now?

* Some women have never snored until they become pregnant. It feels weird and certainly embarrassing, especially when you have never snored before in your whole life. So why now, you wonder! Pregnancy brings many changes to your respiratory system which affects sleep and also causes you to snore. Upto 25-30% of pregnant women snore (so you are not alone!)

* Hormones like estrogen and progesterone increase remarkably during pregnancy giving rise to snoring.

* Anybody can be a candidate for mild to severe snoring during any part of their pregnancy.

Nutrition

Handy foods

* Some foods that we take for granted are in actual fact, quite handy. One such example is potatoes, which are

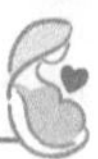

underrated but are actually very nutritious. Try and include them in your diet.

- A potato contains about 3mg of protein, together with calcium, iron, thiamin, riboflavin and niacin; plus seven times as much vitamin C as an apple.

- To cut back on calories, don't fry them. Instead cook them with their jackets by baking or boiling them whole. If you peel them first before cooking, much of the fiber, proteins and vitamins will be lost.

- Milk is another useful food; it is easy to consume and is packed with protein, calcium together with vitamin A and D. Low fat or skimmed milk is preferred over full cream.

- Some of you may not like the taste of milk, so use it on cereals, custards or eat cheese or yoghurt. If you are allergic to milk, ensure you find the right substitutes to provide your body with the nutrients such as calcium which your body needs.

- Your daily needs will be met through your diet alone if you include the following foods on a daily basis: milk or yoghurt, eggs, fish, lean meat, whole grain foods (brown bread, rice or pasta) fresh fruits and vegetables, salads, fruit juices, nuts and dried fruits.

- Calcium can be found in leafy vegetables, dried peas, beans, lentils, and nuts. Calcium supplements also help especially if you are allergic to dairy products; if taken in the compound form you would need 1200mg daily.

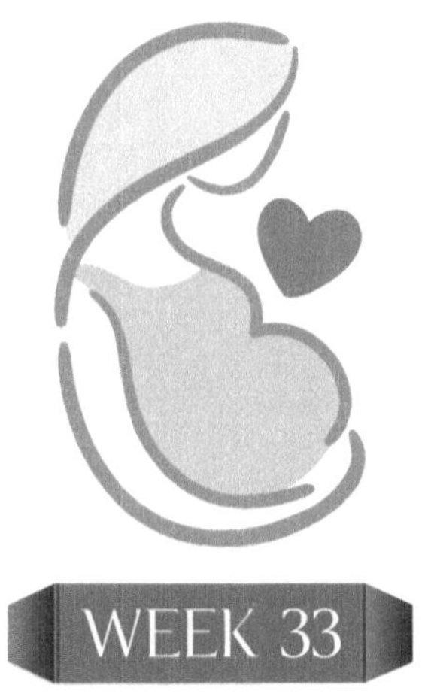

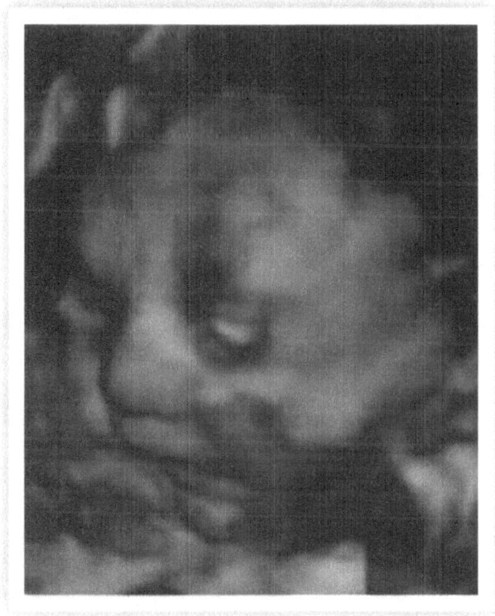

FOETUS AGE 31 WEEKS

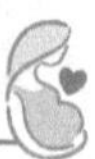

Changes in Baby

- From head to toe, your baby almost measures at 19 inches and weighs about 4.4 pounds.

- All the bones are hardening except for the skull which remains soft and will not completely join - this will enable baby to journey through the birth canal.

- Baby's weight gain is going at a rapid pace, about half a pound a week. The next four weeks will be a period of extraordinary growth.

- The pupils of baby's eyes are now well developed to constrict, dilate and detect light.

- Baby's lungs are now much more developed at this stage.

- Your baby is fast losing the alien, wrinkly look.

Changes in You

- Though you will have bouts of fatigue, you will have bouts of energy as well.

- You may find yourself waddling and bumping into furniture often these days.

- Aches and feeling of numbness in your fingers, wrists and fluid retention are more commonplace - try stretching your hands when you take those frequent breaks.

- You are probably continuing to leak urine, especially when you cough, laugh or sneeze, because your growing baby is pressing on your bladder.

- Your cervix may begin to dilate this week onwards, or sometime in this month - this doesn't mean that you are in labor. Your cervix can dilate week, days or hours before labor begins. Every woman is different.

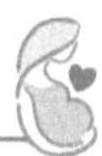

- You will probably have gained a pound a week this month, about 4 pounds in total.

Good to Know

- Fresh foods lose their nutrients rather fast, so it makes sense to have them on the day they are brought. Most of the nutrients are found just under the skin, so eat foods unskinned whenever possible. Root vegetables such as carrots and potatoes should be preferably scrubbed and not peeled. Fruits and vegetables should ideally be eaten in large pieces or whole since they lose vitamins when are sliced or cut.

- Recent studies show that breathing practices encourage the lungs to produce more surfactant, the protein essential for the lung's healthy development.

- The average baby is diapered 7 thousand times before it is potty trained. Newborns need to be changed around 10 times each day and about 7 times a day after 4-6 weeks.

The mucus plug facts

- One sure sign that labor is on the way is when you lose the mucus plug. Tinged with blood or clear in colour, the mucus on your underpants in the last weeks describes this mucus plug. The thick mucus has been blocking the opening to the cervix for a while now.

- Your cervix is the mucus-producing part of your reproductive system.

- The mucus plug functions as a barrier throughout your pregnancy against outside infections.

- This glob of mucus cannot be considered upon as a reliable sign of labor.

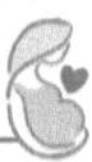

- Dislodgement doesn't necessarily imply that labor is imminent; it could also simply mean that the cervix is going through normal changes.

Wholesome Advice

- Research has shown that women who follow an 8-week regime of pelvic floor exercises during their pregnancy have less urine leakage than women who do not exercise.

- Another tip you can use on food is - never eat food that is past its "sell-by-date" and avoid buying food with damaged packaging such as dents on the cans as the food could be contaminated.

Vaginal Birth After Cesarean (VBAC)

- Once a cesarean, always a cesarean! Not necessarily, although this issue is still under scrutiny because of the uncertainties involved. That explains the low percentage of women opting to give birth vaginally after a cesarean. Many medical practitioners are still divided; some are not totally for it though there are some who are. Vaginal birth after cesarean or VBAC is possible but not without some considerations your doctor will have to take into account.

Your Actions Can Impact Your Baby's Growth

- Pelvic floor exercise - the correct way
- There are things you should avoid when doing pelvic floor exercise. Many people do it the wrong way - the don'ts include:
- Actively contracting the abdominal muscles
- Gripping with the muscles of the legs

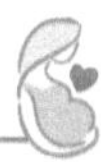

- Tensing or clenching your buttocks
- Holding your breath as you work your pelvic floor
- Tensing your shoulder (you also need to keep your hand relaxed)

Common Concerns

Contraction Stress Test

- Fetal movements translate to fetal well-being. Of course, there are times when the fetus is not active and this does not necessarily imply that the fetus is in trouble. For instance, it is normal for the fetus to move less towards the end of the term because there is less room for movement. There are also situations when due to extra amniotic fluid the mother is not able to feel the movements. To be on the safe side, contact your doctor if you notice movements have decreased considerably. Tests will be carried out to analyze the baby's well being. One such test is the CST or Contraction Stress Test.

Nutrition

- Stress burns energy and uses up vital nutrients such as vitamin C, and minerals such as zinc and magnesium.
- Your dwindling appetite is no help either but it is important to eat food rich in these nutrients as well as the B group of vitamins which are essential to release energy.
- Complex carbohydrates from whole-meal bread which release energy slowly are useful; avoid sugary snacks.
- Raised blood pressure is a common occurrence; a BP

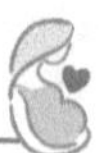

reading greater than 140 over 90 is cause for concern, although it does not show symptoms. First time mums, those carrying twins, very young or older mothers are likely patients of this condition.

- Vitamin C and E have been found to help women combat raised BP. A diet that is low in animal fats and high in fish oil helps to keep the blood thin is recommended.

- Eat plenty of raw fruits and vegetables which are rich in vitamin C and potassium.

- Eat garlic regularly to keep your BP level in check and to improve blood flow in the placenta.

- One tablespoon of sesame or sunflower seeds provide you with the extra calcium and magnesium.

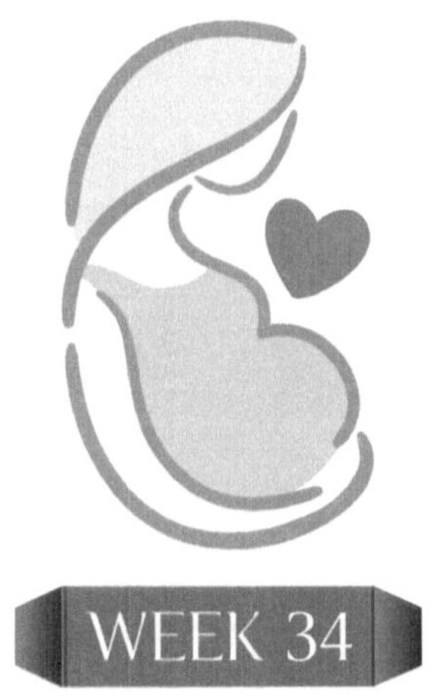

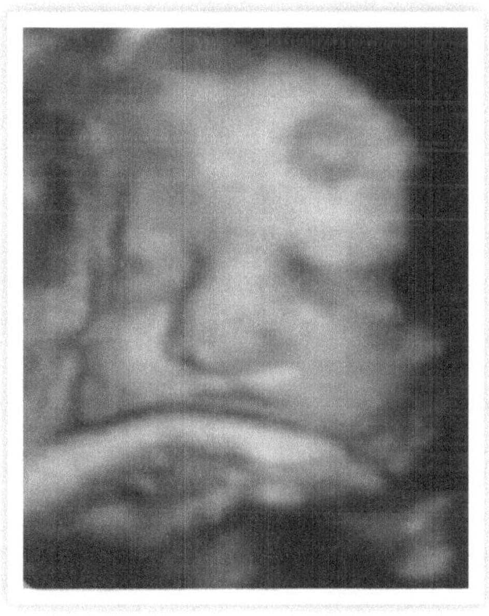

FOETUS AGE 32 WEEKS

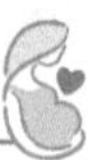

Changes in Baby

* From head to toe, your baby almost measures at 19½ inches and weighs about 5 pounds.

* Vernix or the cheesy coating is getting thicker in preparation for delivery - traces of it can be seen, especially under baby's arm or in the groin area after baby is born.

* The fine baby hair or lanugo had started decreasing for months now; at this stage it is now almost gone!

* Baby's central nervous system is maturing and its lungs are continuing to mature.

Changes in You

* Fatigue has set in once again from those nights of interrupted sleep and physical strain.

* The milk producing glands continue to grow causing your breast size to be bigger.

* You may feel your baby drop sometime this month, settling deeper into your pelvis. As a result you may feel hungrier since baby is no longer putting pressure on your intestines and stomach.

* Heartburn may become less frequent and less severe.

Good to Know

Baby Facts

* Researchers have discovered that babies are probably dreaming as early as week 25 when REM sleep is first observed. Babies may also make faces in response to their dreams.

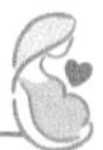

- In twin pregnancies, only one baby may be able to fit into the head down position while its twin fits around as best as it can.

Side Effects of Epidural

- Many are not prepared to hear that epidurals can have side effects. You can vomit, get a bad headache or experience a drop in blood pressure. Sometimes baby's heart rate drops. This temporary problem is rectified with the increased IV, position change and some supplemental oxygen through the nose. The worst happens once the epidural wears off; many women experience the shakes or intense shivering or itching which lasts for less than an hour. Don't panic at this information, but it is important to stay educated.

What is Engagement

- Before engagement, your baby has been floating in the sac above your pelvis.

- Before engagement, you would have had to eat smaller meals more frequently as your baby was occupying too much space; now you are able to handle larger portions.

- You will feel 'lighter' from now and suffer less heartburn; this change is also know as lightening or dropping as your baby drops into the pelvic cavity.

- If this is your first pregnancy, your baby will engage about 2-4 weeks prior to labor.

- If you have had baby before, your baby will not engage until labor actually begins. This is because your uterus muscles have stretched and so there will be less pressure on the baby.

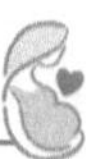

- You will know your baby has engaged when you feel less pressure on your diaphragm and breathing becomes much easier.

Herpes in Pregnancy

- Herpes genitalis is one of the most prevalent sexually transmitted infections. An affected adult shows local symptoms, but affected fetus or newborn can suffer serious infection of the whole body. Herpes in pregnancy rarely results in the fetus acquiring the virus, but a small number of pregnant women do pass on the virus to their babies during labor and delivery. It has been estimated that up to 90% of people don't even know they have herpes. The good part is, a dose of acyclovir taken in the month of delivery is effective in preventing an outbreak during this crucial phase.

Wholesome Advice

- Many hospitals offer walking epidurals which block the sensation of pain without affecting muscles control. This means you can be mobile or at least move your leg so your pushing will be more effective. You can check with your doctor on this.

Pelvic floor exercise during pregnancy

- One of the two groups of muscles that bear the most stress during pregnancy is the pelvic floor muscle. Pregnancy and childbirth weaken the pelvic floor. This is because having a baby puts enormous pressure on these muscles since the muscles have to cope with the weighty uterus and the vaginal stretching that take place during delivery.

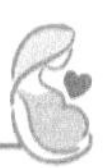

Kegel exercise is most important after delivery to allow the muscles to heal and get back to the pre-pregnancy state. Getting into the habit of doing pelvic floor exercises while pregnant will ensure familiarity with the routine.

Your Actions Can Impact Your Baby's Growth

Position Matters!

* Labor is an active phase and not passive event. The key to a more comfortable labor is position. Being able to assume different positions based on how your body feels will help your labor and generally allow an easier flow of things. Your body will guide you and you should follow these clues. Practicing them ahead of time will help strengthen those muscles and get you geared up mentally as well.

* One such example is to lean forward.

* Learning forward will help tip the baby into your pelvis. This can help lessen the odds of back labor; it can be done by leaning against a birth ball or a person. You can also do it sitting or leaning forward or kneeling, and expect to reap the following benefits:

* Promotes the chances of baby moving into your pelvis

* Induces relaxation

* Can be used in-between or during contractions

Birth Ball

* A good tool to invest in, a birth ball or physiotherapy ball is a fundamentally useful tool for labor. It can be used to ease the strain on your back and bottom, compels you to practice good posture which in turn aids your back. If you don't have one, you can think of getting one now!

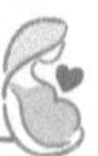

Common Concerns

Please explain the distribution of weight gained in all three trimesters.

* Not very much is gained in the first trimester: Probably 6-11 pounds, most of which is water and materials required for a baby's development. During the 2nd and most of 3rd trimester, you will probably gain about a pound a week. Your weight gain might cease or slow down towards the end of your pregnancy.

Where will the weight go by the end of pregnancy?

* Here is the typical weight breakdown for the end of your pregnancy, quoted in pounds. Any remaining pounds are a general deposit of fat required by the body for breast feeding and energy stores.
  - Baby: 7.5 - 8.5 lbs
  - Amniotic fluid: 2 lbs
  - Increased blood volume: 4-5 lbs
  - Placenta: 2 lbs
  - Breast tissue: 1-2 lbs
  - Uterine muscles: 2.5 lbs
  - Water: 4 lbs
  - Maternal stores: 8 lbs

Nutrition

Omega-3 fatty acids in a gist....

* Omega-3 fatty acids are vital to your diet now. They are important to your baby's proper visual and neurological development. Secondly, through a biochemical mechanism, they delay or prevent the formation of factors

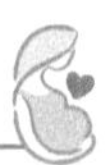

that can lead to premature labor. And finally, they protect your own brainpower. During pregnancy the mother's level of these fatty acids drops considerably - studies indicate that in the final trimester, the mother's brain shrinks by 3%, thus explaining the memory loss. These three factors demonstrate the importance of sufficient omega-3 fatty acids in your diet. Best sources are coldwater fish, flax seed, olive and canola oils. Work on getting 1000 mg of these fatty acids per day.

At a glance...

- Omega-3 fatty acid (the most advantageous version of fatty acids) also called linolenic acid can be found in all seafoods, egg yolk, leaves and seeds of many plants, soybean, nuts; oils such as canola, flaxseed, olive, and walnut, etc.

- Omega-6 fatty acid which is also beneficial can be found in:

    - Nuts including walnuts, peanuts and almonds

    - Seeds such as sunflower seeds

    - Oils such as corn, sunflower and soybean

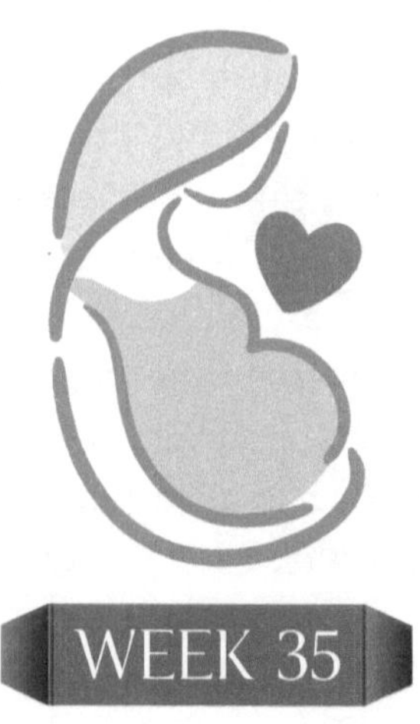

WEEK 35

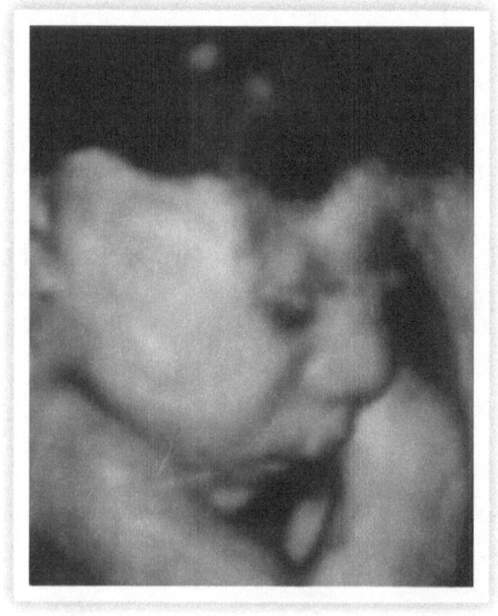

FOETUS AGE 33 WEEKS

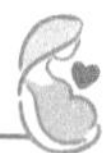

Changes in Baby

* From head to toe your baby almost measures at 20 inches, and weighs about 5½ pounds.

* While your baby will not grow much longer, it still has some weight to gain, about half a pound per week until birth.

* Most of baby's basic physical development is complete - the next few weeks will be spent on putting on weight.

* Fat accumulation is happening especially around the shoulders.

* The next three weeks will likely be your baby's most rapid period of weight gain with weekly gains of up to half a pound.

Changes in You

* From now on, your doctor visits will be on weekly basis.

* The connective tissues in your body are continuing to soften and loosen in preparation for delivery. This is most obvious in your pelvic area.

* Don't stop exercising although you are more prone to muscles and joint injury now.

* Between this week and week 37, you will be checked for Group B Streptococcus (GBS) - a vaginal and rectal culture to check for bacteria.

* You may experience lightening several weeks before delivery or the day labor begins. It is hard to tell when your baby will drop in the pelvis.

Good to Know

Miscellaneous

- 99% of babies born now survive without any major problems.

- According to many podiatrists swollen feet and flat feet are the two most common pregnancy related feet issues.

- There is no set time when breast milk will replace colostrums, though it mostly occurs within 3-5 days of birth.

- Genetics, skin elasticity and weight gain all influence how you will look later. Even if you are small breasted and have breast fed, you will lose some of the elasticity in your breasts. Some degree of post-partum sagging is inevitable.

C-section: Your doctor will most likely suggest surgery if:

- You have had a previous invasive uterine surgery
- You have had previous c-sections
- You are carrying triplets or more
- Your baby is very large
- Your baby is in breech position
- You have placenta previa

When do I go to the hospital?

- Going through the initial pangs of labor in familiar surroundings has its advantages, the main being the comfort of your home when you are anxiety-ridden. Though your apprehension may make you want to rush to the hospital at the first sign you experience, the general advice is the longer you stay at home the better.

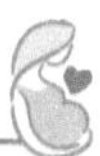

- Being anxious at a time like this is only natural and you would want to be in familiar surrounding that offers comfort. A hospital atmosphere is only going to intensify the unease, and added to that if you arrive too early there is a good chance that you will be sent back home.

Wholesome Advice

- Wear wide shoes and keep your feet elevated whenever you are sitting or lying down. Walk regularly for exercise and avoid salt and fats and drink lots of water. For flat feet, get some good supportive athletic shoes or readymade inserts for your shoes that support and cushion.

How to survive a C-section

- Cesarean is a major abdominal surgery that is becoming quite common these days. The aftercare is important, and that means sufficient rest for speedier recuperation. External scars are the stitches/staples closing the skin and do not form the whole picture. There are layers of muscle and fat, and uterus, which all have been cut during surgery, and there are layers of stitches inside you. If your aftercare has been properly managed, severe pain should not be an issue.

Your Actions Can Impact Your Baby's Growth

The hands and knees position

- This positions (on all fours) works well during the later stages of labor. It is a good position to take in between contractions. It may not stop the contractions but it certainly takes the edge off them. Other benefits include:

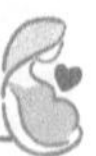

* Helps rotate a baby to the optimal position

* Can provide pain relief especially in case of back labor

* Is a gravity-neutral position, to slow a fast birth

Preparing for a C-section

* Sometimes cesarean birth is best for you and your baby. Though it is normal to have a share of anxieties, almost all mothers and babies recover well after c-section. An operation can be scheduled (planned) or unscheduled (emergency), depending on circumstances and choices made. Both forms involve a series of tasks to be performed prior to the surgery, although some of these steps will be left out totally in an emergency procedure. Some form of anesthesia is always required.

You can squat

* Once your baby is engaged, you can squat. Practice this position before labor in order to reap the benefit. Use a chair to help you learn the position. When in labor you can squat during a contraction and assume a different position between contractions to take off the pressure on your legs. Other benefits include:

* Opens the pelvis more than other positions

* Uses gravity to help pull the baby down

* Can help prevent tears in the perineum

* Works well for pushing

Common Concerns

Is there an ideal position for labor that works for the best?

* The answer is No. There in no one position that works best

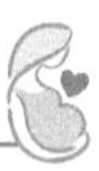

for everyone. With trial and error you will find some positions provide more comfort of pain relief than others. Use the position that works in your favour. On that note, avoid lying on the back totally - this position is often painful and non-productive during labor as it delays the birth process.

How long does labor last?

* The first stage of labor - from the start of contraction to your cervix opening fully - takes an average from 10-14 hours. The second stage is your pushing stage and usually takes about one to two hours but it can feel like ten! The final stage begins when your baby is delivered lasts until the placenta is delivered and on average can take about 15-30 minutes but can be longer.

Nutrition

* A well nourished woman usually develops a healthy placenta. Despite a good supply of nutrients, a baby can become undernourished if the transportation across the placenta is inadequate. Iron is required by the mother to expand her blood volume and by the baby to establish good levels of hemoglobin. If iron levels fall, the efficiency of red blood cells in carrying oxygen is affected and tissues become deficient in energy.

* Zinc is stored in the placenta. High levels of zinc assure a greater birth weight baby.

* Vitamin E, gingko biloba and co-enzyme Q10 are all thought to improve blood supply.

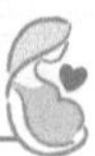

You can improve the efficiency of the placenta in the following ways:

- Eating a balanced diet; good nutrition is vital for a healthy placenta.

- Resting as much as possible - relax the muscles, particularly the abdominals, thereby increasing blood flow to the placenta. Practice relaxation techniques that help eliminate stress and tension from your system.

- Sleeping: Most cell repair and cell growth takes place when you are asleep. So sleep well.

- Giving up work: You should try and stop work by week 32-34. To maintain adequate blood supply, you need to rest in the last 2 months of pregnancy. Stress causes the blood cells to constrict thereby restricting flow. Overwork may cause premature birth and/or low-birth weight baby.

- Problems with the placenta are always linked to raised blood pressure, tobacco, caffeine, alcohol, and overwork and lack of rest. Tests can be conducted to detect placental malfunction; ultrasound measures flow to see if baby's growth is being retarded because of oxygen deprivation.

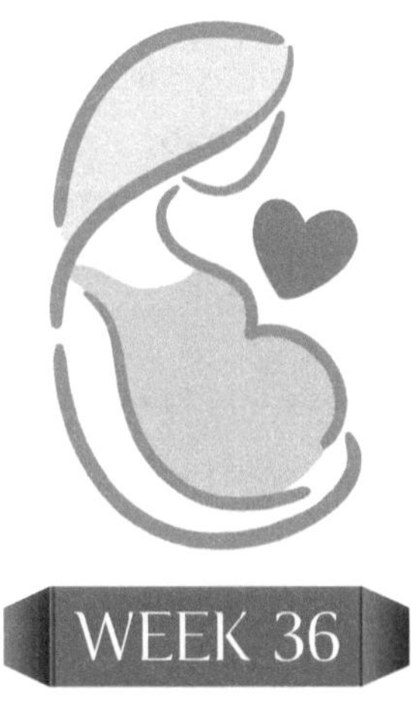

WEEK 36

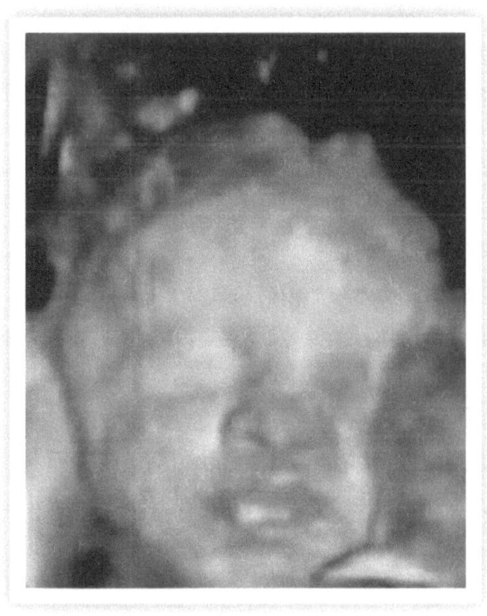

FOETUS AGE 34 WEEKS

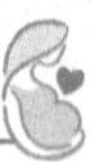

Changes in Baby

- From head to toe, your baby almost measures at 20½ inches and weighs about 6 pounds.

- With just one month to go, all of baby's senses are well-developed.

- All its body parts are sensitive to heat, cold and pressure.

- Baby is shedding most of the downy hair (lanugo) as well as the vernix.

- Baby swallows both sheddings along with other substances, resulting in a blackish mixture called the meconium which will form the content of his first bowel movement.

- Your baby puts finishing touches on its development this week, looking plump and cheeky.

Changes in You

- Starting this week, your doctor will check your cervix for effacement (the cervix stretches and gets thinner) and dilation (opening of the cervix) - signs that you may be going into labor soon.

- You may find yourself consumed with plans for your baby and your new life.

- You may be occupied with thoughts about labor and the pains.

- Your concerns center around everything that is baby-related such as breastfeeding and parenting.

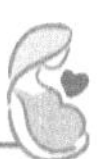

Good to Know

Miscellaneous

- Some C-sections are inevitable no matter how healthy you are, how well you ate or how much you exercised.

- If you delivery vaginally, your vagina is going to be traumatized. Though not permanent, but for few weeks at least, it is going to hurt.

Unplanned C-section

Some problems which can arise and make C-section necessary:

- Your labor stalls - If your cervix stops dilating or your baby stops moving down and your doctor's attempts fail, surgery becomes the alternative.

- Your baby's heart rate becomes a cause for concern.

- Your placenta starts to separate from the wall of the uterus.

- You have an active genital herpes infection.

Recovery from a C-section

- You will be in pain and very sore for a few days - you will certainly need painkillers. The first morning after the operation, a nurse will take out your urinary catheter which is painless. Then she will make you sit up, get up and walk, which is very painful. The first time is usually the worst but after the first 48 hours, you will make rapid progress. The more you move around the better you will feel.

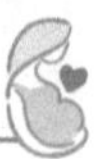

Wholesome Advice

* Your pain medicine causes constipation, so take stool softeners when offered. Pushing is painful after a cesarean.

* Bonding may not always be instant with your newborn - it has got nothing to do with delivery being vaginal or cesarean. So don't feel guilty if you don't bond instantly after your operation.

Your Actions Can Impact Your Baby's Growth

Position Matters: Sitting on a pregnancy ball

* It is easy and comfortable, just like sitting on any chair. The benefit of the ball is that it is much more flexible on your bottom and allows more movement in your pelvis. Besides, it frees your back for massage. Other benefits include:

* Wide variety of uses in labor and birth

* When used in sitting positions, gravity helps the baby descend

* Encourages movement in mother

Sitting on a chair backwards

* Place a pillow over the back of the chair and lean onto it. This position allows you to open your legs and stretch as well as being upright. Other benefits include:

* Use of gravity helps labor progress

* Your legs get to rest

* You get to have back massage from your supporters

* An upright position for giving birth

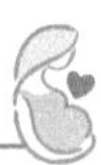

- An upright position will help use gravity to ease and speed the birth process. The most commonly used positions for birth include: Squatting, hands and knees, and leaning forward.

- Each of these positions help to use your body to the fullest.

- These positions also feel better for many women versus reclining positions.

- The position you choose can actually help prevent complications of interventions such as episiotomy.

Common Concerns

How is the placenta delivered?

- After the baby is delivered and the cord is cut, the mother will still have contractions, though not as painful. This part of labor is usually forgotten as the focus goes on the baby. As your placenta separates from the uterine wall, the mother may feel the urge to push or the doctor may instruct the mother to push or may massage your tummy and if all fails your doctor will reach in and take it out. For the curious-minded the placenta resembles a big raw piece of meat with shiny membrane around it.

What is the buzz on episiotomy?

- Episiotomies used to be routine because it was always thought that a clean cut was better than multiple irregular tears. Now it is realized that if you allow the perineum to stretch slowly as the head delivers, you will avoid a significant tear even with a first baby. An episiotomy can lead to excessive tearing all the way through the rectum.

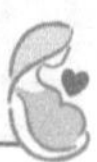

It is also more prone to infection and sexual problems later in life. The vagina is designed to stretch around the baby and then revert to normalcy. Sometimes a small tear is inevitable but it is usually less extensive than an episiotomy and often requires no stitching. There are certain situations that will call for the procedure such as fetal distress, a large baby or a forceps delivery. If you are without an epidural, a local anesthetic will be used.

Nutrition

Iron and anemia

* Many women (more than 90% are slightly anemic before they conceive), particularly those carrying more than one baby, are anemic.

* Anemia occurs if the level of oxygen-carrying hemoglobin in red blood cells drops below normal (when the hemoglobin levels is less than 12.8g/l00 ml blood).

* It is essential to increase your iron intake though prescribed medication to correct iron deficiency anemia before you conceive.

* It is important to have healthy blood during pregnancy in order to prevent complications in labor due to fatigue and to reduce the chances of postnatal depression.

* There are three main causes of anemia: Deficiency in iron, folate or vitamin B12 deficiency; iron deficiency as a result of baby's demands being the most common type.

* If diagnosed with this condition you will be prescribed iron tablets/capsules. Anemia can occur even if you have iron-rich diet since it may be due to lack of B vitamins.

* The following dietary guidelines will be helpful, and since

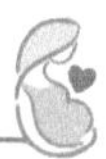

iron cannot be stored in your system, ensure you eat good food sources every day.

- To prevent iron deficiency, eat plenty of green leafy vegetables, pumpkin seeds, cherries, dried apricots, fish and poultry.

- To remedy vitamin B deficiency, eat eggs, milk, cheese, white fish and yeast extract.

- To reduce folate deficiency, eat nuts and raw or steamed green leafy vegetables, wheat germ and pulses.

- To improve iron absorption, consume vitamin C such as fresh orange juice with iron-rich foods which help improve the mineral's absorption.

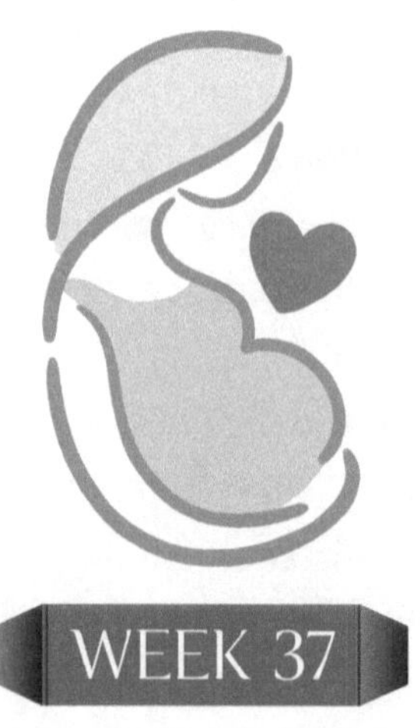

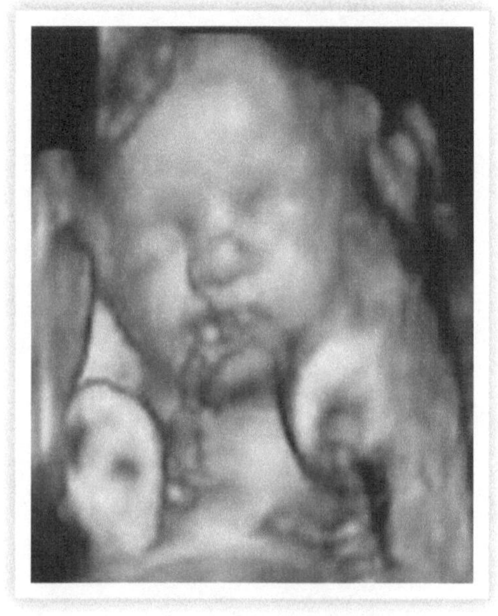

FOETUS AGE 35 WEEKS

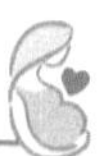

Changes in Baby

- Your baby now weighs about 6½ pounds.

- Weight gain has slowed down to about ½ oz a day; the fat that is being laid down is making your baby become rounder.

- Baby is now considered full term and could be born at any time.

Changes in You

- As your baby settles down into your pelvis, you may have easier time breathing, but start to face bladder discomforts. You will again feel the need to pee frequently.

- You may notice an increase in vaginal discharge now.

- Braxton Hicks contractions may be coming more frequently now and may last longer and be more uncomfortable.

- For most women the next few weeks are a waiting game - use this time to take care of necessary tasks.

Good to Know

1st Stage of Labor

- The first stage is usually the longest and the hardest part of labor. During this stage the cervix gradually opens to allow the baby to make its way down into the birth canal. This stage typically last 10-14 hours with the first baby; in subsequent pregnancies the first stage is likely to be shorter, close to 7 hours.

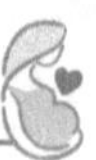

2nd Stage of Labor

- Many women find the second stage easier to cope because they find things under their control more or less. This stage lasts from full dilation until the birth. Once the cervix is completely dilated, baby's head makes its descent through the birth canal. This basically marks the beginning of the second stage.

3rd Stage of Labor

- The final part of labor begins after the baby is born and ends with the delivery of the placenta. Since the mother's entire attention will be on her new baby, she may not even be aware of this part of labor.

Miscellaneous

- Research suggests that it is your baby who triggers labor, producing hormones as a reaction to its cramped surroundings.
- Your baby is now considered full term, meaning it is fully developed and could be born at any time (most first time mothers are late).
- Lightening may occur weeks before the onset of labor or any time right up until the day labor begins.
- The most common description of contractions include periods-like cramps but ten times worse, extreme gas pains, intense pressure, burning or a combination of all these.

Something about labor

- Labor is a unique, intense experience. The common denominator is that childbirth is usually painful.

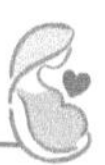

Childbirth is also the bloodiest, messiest and sweatiest event of your whole life. All sorts of fluids and solids, matter and waste matter will be emerge from your system.

Wholesome advice

- The painkiller your take to ease the pain after C-section is constipating; take stool softeners when offered as pushing after the operation is painful.

- In the first few days after delivery, bleeding is especially heavy and messy. You will need jumbo sized pads for a while - as long as you are not soaking a pad every 1-2 hours you are doing just fine. If bleeding increases or there are large clots, this can be a sign of exertion. You need to slow down but despite this if the bleeding doesn't slow down, call your doctor.

Your Actions Can Impact Your Baby's Growth

Pain management after surgery

- After a cesarean, take a small pillow and brace your incision. This will greatly reduced the pain when you are moving about.

- One important concept of pain management, especially after an operation is how you take your medications. If you delay your medicines until you are in pain then you will end up needing more medication for longer period. Instead, take your pain relief medicines at the first sign of pain and then in the next 1-2 days take it by the clock rather than by the symptoms.

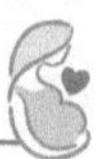

What is stripping the membranes

- Stripping the membranes involves your doctor to separate the amniotic sac from the cervix, with no intention of rupturing the sac as some may believe, but that can happen. Since the bag of water is without nerve endings, it is usually a pain-free experience. Stripping the membranes is known to trigger the labor process within a few days by helping to ripen the cervix. It is however not a form of induction but more a form of stimulation of labor.

Common Concerns

Why does labor hurt more for some than it does for others?

- Sometimes labor hurts more than what is considered normal. This can be due to a complication like back labor. This means your back hurts more due to baby lying in an uncommon position. Labor can hurt more too if there was a previous injury. Sometimes the pain is exaggerated because of external sources such as a vaginal examination or being in positions that are uncomfortable.

How to deal with stitches?

- It takes about 5 days for vaginal stitches to dissolve. Ice packs reduce the swelling. At home, you need to do warm 'sitz' baths where you sit in the tub with water covering just your bums and hips. First, they help with pain and prevent infection and secondly, they force you to sit still and not do anything else which is helpful in your recovery. Do not use toilet paper to clean up, but try to depend on spray bottle filled with water. A cushion for sitting is useful at this point.

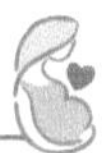

Nutrition

Detoxifying your Body

* Research suggests that the placenta does not block the passage of certain toxins to the baby. To help protect yourself and the baby eat the following foods/nutrients:

* Garlic, onion, bananas, apples and pears to reduce absorption of toxins in general

* Beans, peas and lentils which act as detoxifiers

* B vitamins for general protection

* Vitamin C and zinc to reduce levels of lead in the blood; vitamin E to reduce the risk of lead poisoning and calcium to prevent the absorption of lead.

Antioxidants

* Besides vitamins and minerals, there are other substances that can help prevent disease and promote health - the bioflavonoid. They are potent antioxidants and also give fruits and vegetables their bright colors. They include:
  - Thioesters (garlic, onions, leeks)
  - Terpenes (citrus fruits)
  - Plant phenols (grapes, strawberries, apples)
  - Carotenoids (carrots, yams, sweet potatoes, watermelons)
  - Lutein (tomatoes)

* The most nutritious fruits and vegetables are the fresh variety; frozen and canned varieties are acceptable too. As long as you are eating the recommended amount of fruits and vegetables, you are getting the bioflavonoid that you and your baby need.

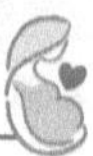

A word on Folic Acid

- All women of childbearing age who are capable of becoming pregnant should consume folic acid every day. The recommended dose is:

    - 400 mg a day for all women of childbearing age

    - 600 mg a day for pregnant women

    - 500 mg a day for lactating mothers

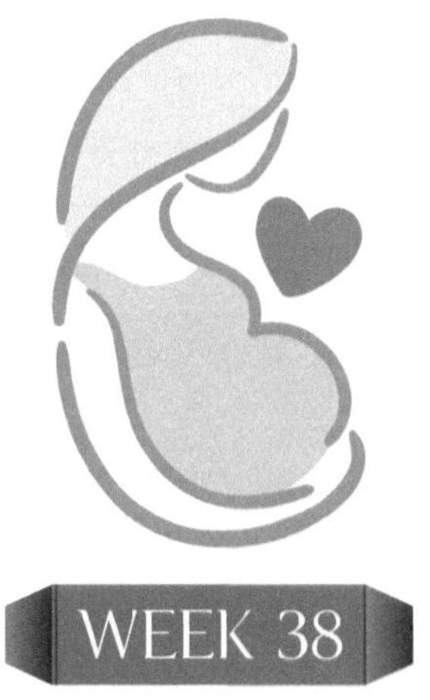

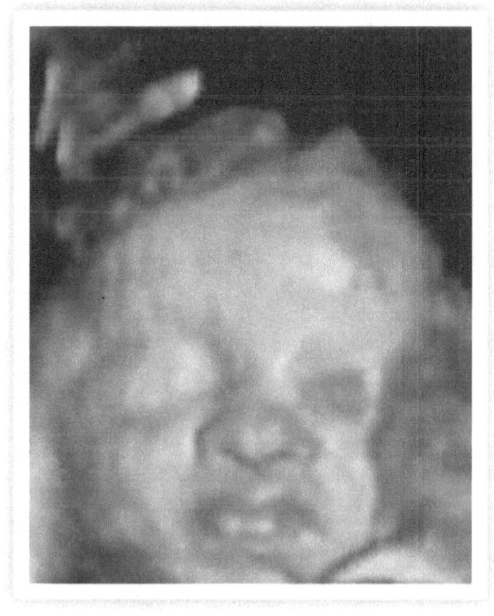

FOETUS AGE 36 WEEKS

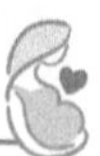

Changes in Baby

- Your baby now weighs anywhere between 6-8 pounds and measures at about 14 inches from crown to rump. (Notably, boys tend to be heavier than girls).

- Baby's organs have matured and are ready for life outside the uterus.

- This month your baby has worked on managing the complicated tasks of breathing, digesting, keeping the right heart rate and eating.

Changes in You

- Swelling in your legs and ankles is normal during this time but not in your hands or face.

- Your digestive system remains slowed this month because of the hormones, unless your baby drops into your pelvic (lightening).

- Your uterus will complete its expansion; at term, it will extend from your pubic area to bottom of your rib cage.

Good To Know

Miscellaneous

- Big babies do happen to small people.

- It is very common to have bowel movement or to urinate while having a contraction or pushing.

- Neither you nor your baby will feel a thing when the cord is clamped.

- Your vagina is going to be traumatized for a few weeks if you deliver vaginally.

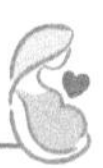

- Lochia is a mixture of blood, mucus, and placenta leftovers that your body will expel for about 6 weeks post delivery.

Symptoms after birth:

- Fatigue you experience now, will be intense because of physical and emotional changes you went and are going to go through.

- Hemorrhoids caused by strain of pushing.

- Frequent urination, as your body needs to rid itself off all the extra fluid. Also, your bladder may have trouble emptying fully because it became stretched out.

- Cramps and contractions occur for a few weeks especially if you are breastfeeding. Your uterus is returning to its normal size over a period of 6 weeks.

- Hair loss will persist until your hormones normalize.

- You may not always make it to the bathroom. After a vaginal birth especially with a big baby, the changes to your bladder and pelvic floor muscles are the causes.

Wholesome Advice
Accept any help that is offered because you will need it.

- The truth is, it is very confusing for many first-time pregnant women to know when they are in labor or when labor is starting. Don't feel embarrassed if you have to check with your doctor often.

Your Actions Can Impact Your Baby's Growth
Your Labor Bag

- Now is probably the right time to pack a basic kit for the birth and afterwards. You will need:

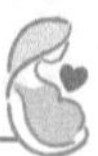

- Nightdresses with front opening
- Maternity bras
- Breast pads
- Sanitary towels
- Toiletries - toothbrush & toothpaste, brush & comb, face cream, shower gel, shampoo, make-up, mirror, perfume, etc.

Your baby will need:

- Nappies
- Blanket
- Suitable clothes 2-3 sets
- Car seat - you must fit a suitable baby seat to the car in which baby will travel

The extras:

- An extra pillow
- A thick pair of socks
- A hot water bottle for pain relief
- Massage oil
- A box of tissues

Learn to recognize the real thing

- True labor is defined as regular painful contractions that cause cervical dilation.
- Often it can be difficult for you to tell if you are in true labor. Signs of true labor are:
- After timing the contractions, you notice them coming consistently and closer in pace.

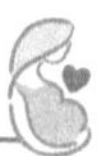

- Each contraction lasts anywhere from 30 to 70 seconds and gets longer.

- Your contractions do not ebb even after you change your activity.

- The contractions starts in the lower back radiate to the front.

- Your water breaks.

- Usually, once you find that you have been having painful contractions that seems to occur every 5 minutes for 2-3 hours, it is fair to consider yourself in labor. However, this doesn't mean you are ready to deliver. There are still many hours before you would be offered an epidural.

Reasons for amniotomy

- By far, the most common reason for amniotomy is to induce labor or speed up contraction in prolonged labors. Prostaglandin from the amniotic fluid is released which strengthens and increases the frequency of uterine contractions.

- To better scrutinize the fetal heartbeat by placing strategically an internal fetal electronic monitor on baby's scalp. This equipment will reliably record baby's heartbeat.

- To check the presence of meconium in the fluid, an indication of fetal distress, by observing the color of amniotic fluid. Immediate action can be taken to suction the contents of baby's bowel should it be necessary.

- Mostly the sac tends to break on its own during the second stage of labor but infrequently baby can be born with an intact sac which must be quickly broken to allow baby to breathe.

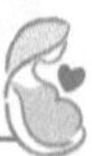

Common Concerns

Biophysical Profile

* Also known as BPP, this is a non-invasive procedure that evaluates baby's well being with the aid of a non-stress test combined with an ultrasound. Again, this test is conducted in the later part of pregnancy to check on baby's well-being, especially in situations when the mother has pre-existing medical problems, in mothers who develop conditions in the course of the pregnancy or pregnancies that go beyond 40 weeks. The ultrasound is used to monitor body movements, breathing, amniotic fluid levels and muscle tone of the baby.

How will I know when my 'water' sac breaks?

* Many women don't even realize that it has happened because it can be very unobvious. What you may feel is a warm trickle of liquid. You could also hear a pop sound and feel gush or a trickle. You may get confused between 'water' breaking and your bladder. The wise thing to do is to put on a sanitary pad and lie down for 20 minutes or so. When you stand up and you feel another tickle or gush then chances are your 'water' did break.

How will I know if the head has engaged?

* The most obvious change you will notice is your bump looking lower than it did and the kicks you felt in the ribs are less. You may need to pee more often. Also termed lightening, your doctor will confirm this event by an external examination.

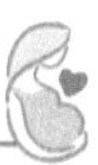

Nutrition

* During the last few weeks of pregnancy, you should build on the preceding months of healthy eating so that you are prepared for the rigors of labor.

* Vitamin K is needed for blood clotting, preventing hemorrhaging and helps to heal the placental site. It is derived naturally from the mother's gut and supplemented from food such as broccoli, beans, spinach, avocado, cabbage, cauliflower, lettuce, etc.

* An infant depends on its mother for vitamin K; before birth via the placenta and after birth through breast milk. (Babies may be given vitamin K orally at birth).

* Zinc is another important mineral required for hormone production and healing after birth.

Energy production

* To maintain energy level, you need to keep your blood sugar level constant by eating complex carbohydrates, which break down gradually and release sugar content slowly.

* Eat lots of vegetables, grains and pulses to stock up on complex carbohydrates during the two weeks before birth.

* Additionally, enzymes are needed; these are dependent on vitamins and minerals. Enzyme deficiency will prevent you from maximizing your energy potential. To convert glucose into energy you need:

* *The B group of vitamins (B1, B2, B4, B6, B12).*
Sources: Meat, poultry, milk, eggs, vegetables, pulses, nuts and whole grains.

* *Vitamin C:* Sources: Citrus fruits, tomatoes, broccoli

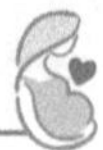

- *Choline:* Sources: Eggs, fish, soy beans, whole grains, nuts, pulses

- *Calcium & Magnesium:* Sources: Cheese, milk, beans, nuts, raisins

- *Chromium: Sources:* Potatoes, wholemeal bread, eggs, chicken

- *Co-enzyme Q10:* Sources: Meat, fish, eggs, soy beans, spinach, broccoli

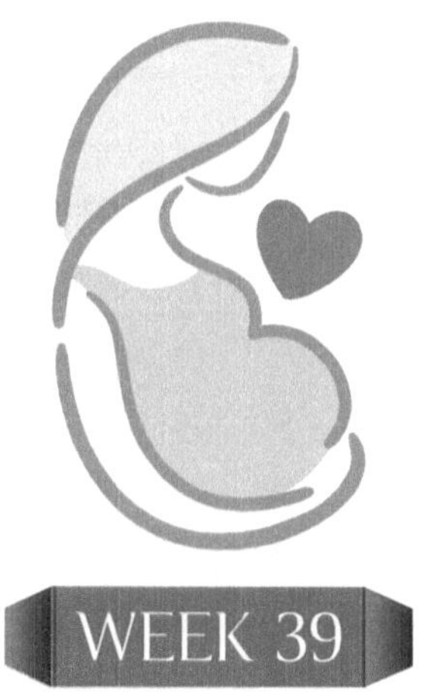

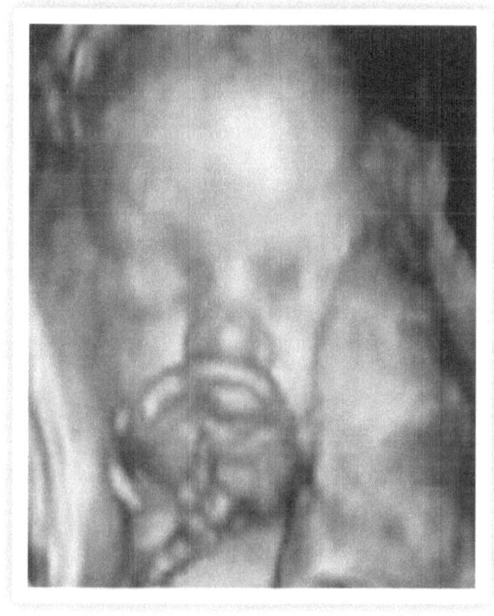

WEEK 39

FOETUS AGE 37 WEEKS

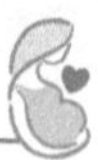

Changes in Baby

- Your baby now weighs between 7-7½ pounds, although it is normal for babies to weight from 6-9 pounds.

- Your growing baby sheds the outer layers of its skin as new skin forms underneath.

- Babys head is still its largest part and hence best that baby is born headfirst.

- The placenta continues to offer protection with antibodies against harmful bacteria and viruses.

- Your baby's arms and legs are in a flexed position.

Changes in You

- This week Braxton Hicks contractions get stronger and more forceful, preparing your cervix for labor.

- On the downside, sleep is a problem and your mood swings are not any help.

- At your weekly visits, your doctor will do an abdominal examination to check baby's growth and position; an internal examination to check the state of the cervix.

- Treat yourself by visiting the spa for a brief session of manicure/pedicure.

Good to Know
Miscellaneous

- Your baby will swallow its lanugo along with other secretions and store them in its bowels.

- At 51 cm or 20 inches long, the umbilical cord is as long as your baby from head to toe.

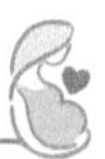

- Pregnancy hormones produced by your body may cause the breast in both newborn boy and girls to be swollen at birth and even produce tiny amount of milk.

- The hardest phase of labor is the shortest.

- A full bladder or bowel can stand in the way of baby's progress down the birth canal.

Epidural Anesthesia - The pros & the cons

- Epidural anesthesia is the most common form of pain relief for laboring women, and they resort to it for valid enough reasons. One such reason being the wish to conserve their physical and emotional energies for later after their baby arrives. Secondly, labor can be truly a painful experience for many, much beyond their endurance. And finally, majority of women want to be active participants during the birthing process. Many women embrace this form of pain relief for the benefit it offers, but it is good to be aware of the drawbacks irrespective of the decision you will make.

Wholesome Advice

- Bonding with your newborn can take several days, weeks and even months. You are just so relieved that labor or your C-section is over. It's okay - you will bond later.

- An IV line should be inserted into the arm you use least, as you will be left with a bruise for a while. If you are right handed ask for the left and vice versa.

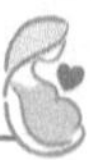

Your Actions Can Impact Your Baby's Growth

If you must be induced...

Here are the options used if induction becomes necessary:

* Amniotomy is the process where your doctor will break the sac. This sac won't break until you are well into labor. With induction, an instrument will go up into your vagina and through the cervix to make a hole in the membrane. Usually painless but a little uncomfortable, the rupture allows the water to flow out and labor pains to begin.

* Stripping the membranes is a procedure usually done in the doctor's office where your doctor will insert a finger into the cervix and try to separate the membrane from where it is attached to the wall of the uterus. The discomfort comes more from the vaginal examination than anything else.

* Synthetic hormones also trigger labor. The mother will be given Oxytocin or Pitocin via a IV line. Once these agents are in your bloodstream your uterus swings into action. These hormones work by mimicking normal labor.

Common Concerns

My concern is why women aren't induced as soon as they pass their due dates?

* There is a good reason for this. If mother and baby are not ready for labor, all the Pitocins (the synthetic version of oxytocin given through IV) in the world will not start the labor. For induction to work smoothly the cervix has to be as ripe as possible and until that happens all a doctor will do is to monitor the mother closely.

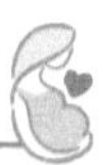

Is it true that I won't be able to eat or drink anything during labor?

* Laboring women are not supposed to ingest anything during labor because digestion shuts down during this time. Anything consumed at this point will just sit there and later cause you digestive problems or make you feel nauseous or have diarrhea. Another reason why foods and liquids are off limits, is in the event of an emergency and when general anesthesia is used, the stomach remnants will cause the mother to vomit and choke. All said and done, laboring for hours is a tedious process that is energy-consuming.

Long labor

* A long labor though normal, can be difficult to handle. It is especially common in first time pregnancy, with over 80% labors lasting beyond 12 hours without medical intervention. Not only is it exhausting, it makes the laboring woman feel unaccomplished. Having said that, it is difficult to quantify the total length of labor before it is considered prolonged.

Nutrition

A word on Calcium, Magnesium and Zinc

These three minerals are essential for your baby.

* Calcium significantly reduces your risk of developing preeclampsia, which is more prevalent in women pregnant for the first time.

* Magnesium helps to prevent premature labor by minimizing uterine contractions. It also lowers your

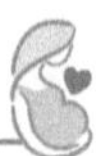

baby's risk of cerebral palsy or mental retardation after birth because it provides protection to the developing nervous system.

- Zinc is vital for the healthy development of your baby's nervous system. It also reduces the incidences of infection during pregnancy.

- These minerals also reduce the occurrences of heartburn, leg cramps and insomnia.

- Women lack calcium, primarily because generally adults drink inadequate amounts of milk. If you avoid milk because of being intolerant, then choose lactose free milk. 2 grams of calcium per day is sufficient; this can be obtained from dairy foods, calcium rich foods such as salmon, broccoli and tofu.

- If you choose to include calcium supplements, then your best bet is either calcium carbonate or calcium citrate for best absorption. Calcium carbonate is the most concentrated and economical form of calcium. Finally, calcium is absorbed the best when taken with food.

- Your target for magnesium should be 800 mg. Dairy foods are a rich source; other food options are fruits and vegetables (bananas, beans, spinach, avocados) and grains foods (oatmeal and brown rice).

- For zinc your goal is 30 mg per day. Protein foods such as meat and eggs, dairy food and grains provide you with zinc that you require.

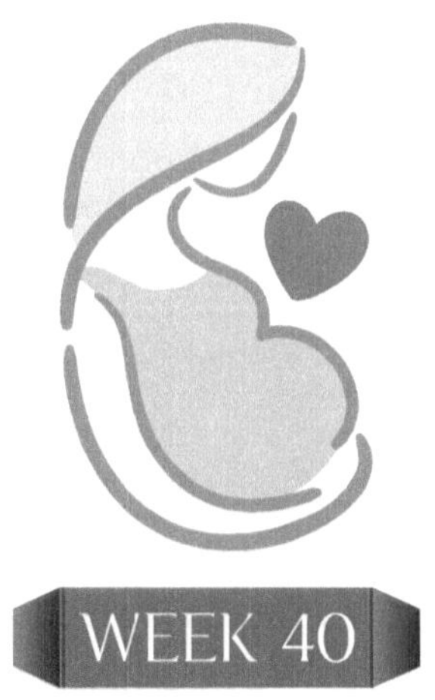

WEEK 40

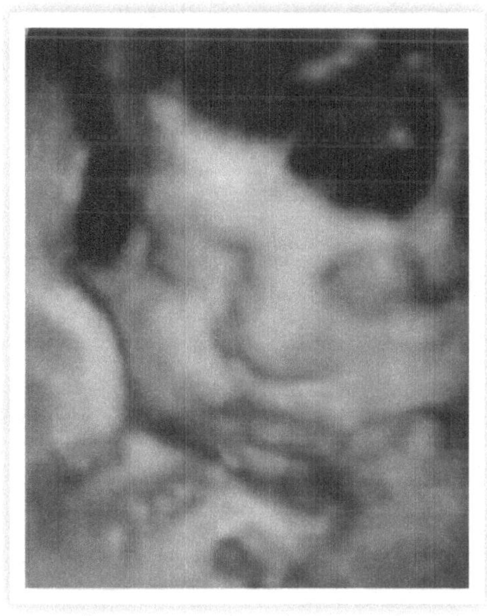

FOETUS AGE 38 WEEKS

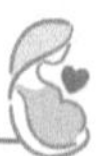

Changes in Baby

* At 40 weeks, over 95% of babies are head-down in the uterus and will be born this way.

* The average weight of a newborn at term is about 3.4 kg, although anything between 2.5-4 kg is considered normal.

* From 37 or 38 weeks, your baby may not have gained much weight.

* Only about 5-6% babies are born on the due date. The majority are born after 40 weeks.

* There is about one liter of amniotic fluid surrounding your baby, which at this point is milky in consistency due to the lanugo mixed in it.

Changes in You

* You may have lost a little weight in the final couple of weeks. Your weight gain has slowed down or stopped from about week 37. So you may lose about 900-1.4 kg in the last few weeks.

* You will still have a week or two before you were considered 'late' since full term is considered anywhere from 37 to 42 weeks.

Good to Know

Baby Facts

* Equipped with over 70 different reflexes, your baby is ready to start its new life outside the uterus.

* The placenta at this point is roughly one-sixth of the size of the baby.

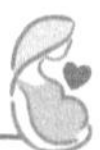

- The umbilical cord is about the same length as the baby.
- Baby's immune system takes time to fully mature and will develop slowly over the first few years of its life. The myelin sheath that coats the nervous system also needs to mature and will be complete when your child turns about two years old.

Mummy Facts

- After delivery, most women lose about 12 pounds immediately (7-9 pound baby, 1-2 pounds placenta and about 1 pound of blood and amniotic fluid). The weight loss continues as all the extra fluid will need to be flushed out. Expect more urine and perspiration than usual in the days after birth. By the end of the 1st week you will lose about 4 pounds of water weight (This of course depends on how much water was retained during pregnancy).
- An over-distended bladder can cause urinary problems and make it harder for the uterus to contract, thereby causing more bleeding and pains. If there is a problem with peeing, a catheter will be placed in the bladder to release urine. A catheter will be placed for women who have undergone a C-section for some hours post delivery.

Wholesome Advice

- If baby blues hit you, know that it is treatable; know that you are not alone.

Symptoms of baby blues:

- Weepiness or crying for no apparent reason
- Impatience
- Irritability

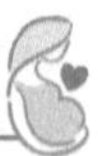

- Restlessness
- Anxiety
- Fatigue
- Insomnia (even when the baby is sleeping)
- Sadness
- Mood changes
- Poor concentration

Your Actions Can Impact Your Baby's Growth

Post Delivery: Dos and Don'ts

When can I Exercise?

- Short walks and simple exercises within days after birth are generally considered fine. If you had a cesarean, wait till your doctor okays it.

When can I start dieting?

- Not until the six weeks are up for sure. You need time to recover from labor and delivery. After this time frame, crash dieting is ruled out if you are breastfeeding.

When can I go back to work?

- 6 weeks following a vaginal birth and 2 months after a C-section. If you are in a rush to resume work, make sure you don't tax yourself with long hours. Many women take several months to heal physically and/or emotionally to feel fit for work.

5 Pointers for New Mothers

- Don't crash diet or skip meals: you need enough calories and nutrients to recover from childbirth to maintain your energy level and milk supply if you are breastfeeding.

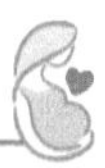

- Focus on healthy foods: eat foods that are rich in protein, calcium and iron.

- Stay hydrated: drink at least 8-12 glasses of water a day.

- You may need supplements: you still need a healthy balanced diet which means good eating habits and the supplements your doctor prescribes.

- Avoid irritants, especially if you are breastfeeding: cut back on caffeine as this irritates newborns. In some cases of allergy, other foods such as cow's milk, nuts etc. should be eliminated following your doctor's advice.

Common Concerns

When will the cord be cut after the birth?

- This depends on the method and circumstances of delivery. If there was a surgery the cord will be clamped immediately. In vaginal births you have the choice of leaving the cord intact until it stops pulsating.

What triggers labor?

- The miracle of birth is still a medical mystery though labor is plainly defined as a series of uterine contractions that opens the cervix for birth. Somehow, the baby's system coupled with the mother's hormones and the placenta all play a role in triggering labor. The current understanding is that labor begins when hormones (prostaglandins) of the mother are produced in large amount which in turn cause contractions to become stronger. These contractions in turn increase the production of prostaglandins further and the cycle progresses into labor.

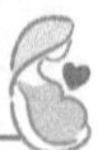

Nutrition

- How you feel emotionally and physically after a C-section will depend largely on whether you had an elective (planned) or an emergency section (rushed into theatre because of concerns about you or the baby). The latter can leave you feeling shocked and emotional and you are more likely to have had a general anesthetic.

Possible Problems:

- Side effect of the anesthetic

- Fatigue and tearfulness

- Infection

- Insufficient lactation

Key tips:

- Get as much rest as possible to aid healing and recuperation.

- Allow yourself time to recover properly and do not attempt to do too much.

- Eat a healthy diet, especially zinc-rich food as this will help you heal faster.

- A good diet is important following C-section. Take a daily multivitamin and eat plenty of foods rich in vitamin C (citrus fruits and broccoli), iron and zinc (fish, poultry and whole grain) to encourage your body to fight infection and aid iron absorption, to help your wound heal and to prevent anemia (if you lost a lot of blood). In addition, take energy rich drinks and light meals or snacks regularly. Take a DHA supplement if you are breastfeeding.

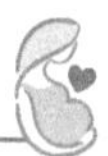

- *Note:* If you develop fever, chills, extreme fatigue, flu-like symptoms or your wound is inflamed and does not seem to be healing properly, you may have an infection. Consult your doctor.